LIVING
WHOLE BODY
HEALH

Dr. Timothy Weeks

Supplement

Fulvic/Humic Minerals

PUBLISHED BY KDP PUBLISHING

Copyright © 2018 by Dr. Timothy Weeks

Book design: Timothy Weeks

Illustrations: Timothy Weeks

Library of Congress Cataloging-in Publication Data

ISBN: 9781973129639

Living Whole Body Health / Timothy Weeks - 1st ed

1 - Nutrition 2. Mind and body therapies

Dedicated to:

The billions worldwide suffering with chronic disease and being deceived by the medical industry. I pray this book gives you hope.

Acknowledgements:

-Thank you to all the holistic healers who laid out the foundations of this book. Thank you for putting your love of humanity before your aspirations of greed. You are my inspiration.

-Thank you Mom and Dad for believing in me, loving me, and being seekers of truth.

-Thank you Ali, my beautiful wife, for enduring my endless pursuit of Whole Body Health and loving me through the process.

-Thank you Frank Revy for your time helping me write this book. Without the thousands of hours spent talking to you and multiple trips to Costa Rica, this book would have never happened.

-Thank you Jeff Weeks and Craig Ihms for helping me edit this book.

-Thank you Amanda and Brian Weeks, my siblings, for joining me in the Chiropractic profession. It has not been easy, but the road to truth never is.

-Thank you Ben for helping me see the golden pathway in life.

-Thank you to everyone reading this—together we can change the world.

CONTENTS:

SECTION 1: The Whole Body Health Paradigm   1

A TESTIMONIAL - Daniel "Prasad" Moss   1

FOREWORD - Douglas Weeks M.D.   3

CHAPTER 1: Broken to Whole Body Health   6

CHAPTER 2: The Truth   13

CHAPTER 3: The Breaking Point   20

CHAPTER 4: Life is About Making Choices   31

CHAPTER 5: Rockefeller Medicine   50

CHAPTER 6: The Shift to the Sugar Age   56

CHAPTER 7: The Solution to the Sugar Age   71

SECTION 2: The Manual   **78**

CHAPTER 8: Introduction to Section 2   78

CHAPTER 9: Healing the mind   83

CHAPTER 10: The Carbohydrate Reset   95

CHAPTER 11: Minerals and Vitamins   121

CHAPTER 12: Digestive Dominos   138

CHAPTER 13: Stomach Domino   141

CHAPER 14: Liver and Gallbladder Domino   149

CHAPTER 15: Small Intestine Domino   156

CHAPTER 16: Colon Domino   173

CHAPTER 17: Oxygen   186

CHAPTER 18: Movement   204

CHAPTER 19: Water Safety   220

CHAPTER 20: Living Structured Water   230

CHAPTER 21: The Sun's Healing Fire   239

CHAPTER 22: The Nervous System   251

CHAPTER 23: Cannabis   260

CHAPTER 24: Conclusion   270

SECTION 3: Appendix   **272**

Appendix A: Phase I Foods   272

Appendix B: Week of Meals (examples)   275

Appendix C: Recipes   278

Appendix D: Allergy Elimination Instructions   288

Appendix E: Liver Flush Instructions   291

Appendix F: Coffee Enema Instructions   293

References: **295**

SECTION 1: THE WHOLE BODY HEALTH PARADIGM

A TESTIMONIAL:

There I was waiting in line to hear yet another doctor speak. I remember standing outside the hall thinking to myself that this session, like hundreds of others I have attended, would surely be a waste of time. I knew my fibromyalgia was incurable and wanted to spare myself from getting my hopes high only to crash again into despair and disappointment. I figured this doctor, like all the others, had little to offer. My skepticism was real.

For 20 years, since being diagnosed with fibromyalgia at the age of 17, I've visited with healers from all over the globe from Jordan to India. I had previously given up and accepted the fact that this miserable condition was my fate. I had quit even trying to explain the condition to the people in my life. A healthy person simply cannot understand the ceaseless chronic pain and constant fatigue I was experiencing.

I decided to focus on the good fortunes of my life, which was my family, friends, and community. But here I was in line again. I was about to turn around and walk away when something happened. We were having some small talk when suddenly I heard Ben, Dr. Tim's friend and assistant, say something that shocked me with hope to the core. Ben said, "I used to have fibromyalgia."

Now, you must understand that for the past 20 years of chronic pain and suffering, I never heard anyone talk about fibromyalgia in the past tense. "I used to have fibromyalgia..." What a strange thing to say.

I lingered after the session, still skeptical, but with an intense feeling of urgency. Without really knowing what I was getting myself into, I looked Dr. Tim in the eyes and asked him, "Can you help me?"

He told me he could and became my guide for 21 days. He wrote this book for me during the 21 day period as my own personal healing manual. Now he's sharing it with you. His insights and knowledge in this book work. The healing is real.

If you have fibromyalgia or any other disease and are reading these words, I know how you feel. I know what it feels like to lose hope of healing and accept a life of pain. I know because I had given up hope years ago. I say to you now and know this for a fact: There is a way out. I am living proof of it. I used to have fibromyalgia. Listen to Dr. Tim's words and take them to heart. Then raise yourself up one more time and really go for it. Soon you too will be living whole body health.

—Daniel "Prasad" Moss

FOREWORD—Dr. Douglas Weeks

It is with a whole lot of pride, a bit of regret, and much happiness that I write the forward to this book.

Pride—because Dr. Tim has been able to take a long look at medicine and communicate it in this book. He described what it has been, what it is today, and what it can become. As a physician myself, I am very proud of him.

Regret—because Dr. Tim, my son, is the 6th consecutive generation of doctors in the family, dating back to the early 1800s and, as far as I know, the only one who has communicated his view of medical care and published it. Yes, his great-great grandfather, Oliver Weeks M.D., was wounded in the Civil War and subsequently became a physician, but didn't write about it. His grandfather, Frank Weeks M.D., kept a diary during his years in the Pacific Theater as a surgeon during World War II, but never published it for the benefit of others. I planned to write a book about my 20 years as an emergency physician, and subsequent transition to Integrative Medicine, as I learned that drugs and surgery are not the way to return one to health, but haven't done it.

Happiness—because Dr. Tim has communicated his ideas and plan for health to many who are hurting, losing hope for their health, and disappointed at standard medical treatment. If you follow his precepts, you cannot help but improve and get on the path to real healing for the body and mind. Most of all, you will be happy because you will achieve independence for your health. Instead of sitting passively, waiting for a doctor's verdict and another prescription for another drug, you can actively improve on your own.

I have always felt that truth is like a castle, up on a hill. As one tries to get to it, one encounters all sorts of

3

obstructions—barbed wire, a moat, land mines—all trying to making it hard to get there. The truth in medicine is the same: It is very hard to get to, for the reasons that Tim elucidates in these pages—politics, policies started by Rockefeller, medical associations, government agencies, drug companies, lobbyists, and all those who are more concerned with money and self-interest than the health of their fellow citizens. As you read these pages, your eyes will be opened as truth will be revealed to you.

I have long felt that if you really understand a subject, you should be able to communicate it to others so that they might understand it with minimal effort. Yet it is very hard for the patient to understand their problems because doctors obfuscate it with their shielding of white coats and esoteric language. I am convinced that many doctors themselves don't really understand the way the body works and the way to health. They don't understand how cholesterol works in our bodies—they just want to knock it down because of a myth that it is all bad. They don't understand the role that bacteria play in our health nor how the gut works—they just want to knock it out with an antibiotic. Since they don't understand these things, they resort to training by drug companies and the "learned physicians" who are paid by the drug companies to just attack problems, not nourish and balance the body so it might heal itself. But Dr. Tim has studied extensively and learned. Now he presents these concepts in a clear, understandable way, using humor, analogies, and case reports so you can walk away with usable knowledge.

He makes you the managing partner in your healthcare, but makes no bones about it—if you want to achieve your goals, you are going to have to change some things and it probably won't be easy at first. There are no quick, passive fixes. You will have to eat right, drink good water, detoxify, and avoid sugar and other toxic substances. The reward will be beyond your expectations and you will be set free. As he writes in the first page of his book, "A healthy person has many dreams, a sick person has but one." Your dreams can be restored with your health.

This is a book you will want to read, read again, and then keep as a reference. As his father, I know Dr. Tim very well and I know his goal is not to just throw a book out there nor try to entice you to buy something. He truly wants to see you healthy and strong and happy. Enjoy it and employ it.

—Douglas Weeks M.D.

I - BROKEN TO WHOLE BODY HEALTH

"Life is short, the art long." —Hippocrates

A healthy person has many dreams, a sick person has but one. A health crisis is a great motivator—it's probably what led you to this book. It means that some symptom or condition has pained you enough that you're finally deciding to do something. It means you dream of a better life, free from illness.

Just like you, I was looking for answers years ago when my health began to fail me, and just like you are about to, I found the answers.

A common definition of insanity is expecting a different result upon repeating the same action. Perhaps you're reading this book because you're realizing that change is required. Most likely your symptoms are awakening in you the truth that no matter what you do, every year you feel worse and your overall quality of life is failing. You might realize the only recent gains in your life are weight, anxiety and pain. You are finally ready to heal.

Regardless of how much you believe in your current doctor or health regimen, results are the only thing that matters. Lack of results must dictate a new approach. At least this is how I felt when I got sick and found no help from the current health system. I eventually lost faith in doctors and decided to look for a better approach.

Each of us will have health challenges in life. What matters is not how or when we will be affected, but rather how we deal with it. Do we accept our new fate or do we strive for better? This is the most important question you can possibly ask yourself.

Here is a short story of my health breaking point and how I discovered a healing formula and cured myself:

When I was nine years old, it was the best year of my young life yet. It was summer break and I got to ride my bike to basketball camp. I loved playing basketball. One day riding back home from camp, a car ran me over.

The elderly driver did not see me at the crosswalk, nor realize she hit me. As she drove away my body got stuck underneath the moving car. I tumbled, rolled, bounced, and was dragged for 50 yards underneath her car before I was finally spit out onto the road.

Amazingly, my life was spared, though 90% of my skin was covered in wounds and abrasions, and my left leg and ankle were shattered.

I felt like my body was broken. I spent three weeks in the hospital, bedridden, trying to recover. My bones eventually healed and my wounds became scars. To the outside observer, it seemed that I had mended, but to me something was wrong I could not articulate. I no longer felt good. Not able to put my finger on it, I lived with a change I did not understand.

As time went on, my health deteriorated. I remained active, but over the next four years I broke my right arm four times and each of my front four teeth often doing simple activities. My bones had become incredibly weak.

My M.D. father prescribed medications to try to alleviate my worsening ADHD. I developed severe, embarrassing acne. Frequent colds and flus were my norm. In seventh grade my feet went flat; the pain from walking distances was barely alleviated by the special arches prescribed by a podiatrist.

At the end of eighth grade my parents decided to hold me back a year, feeling I wasn't physically or emotionally ready for high school. I felt inadequate.

When I got to high school, I kept Pepto-Bismol in my locker and my car for my relentless stomach pains. I collected more injuries. My best friend and basketball teammate, also named Tim, told me that I had the worst injury list of anyone he'd ever seen. While playing basketball, I regularly sprained both my ankles. My left shoulder dislocated over 100 times, often forcing hospital visits. It got so bad that I couldn't lift my arm above my head without it going out of socket. It started dislocating during my sleep, when I put my arm around a friend for a picture, and while playing frisbee.

Despite all this I pushed on, did my best, and was accepted to Ohio University's pre-med program in 1998. It was my freshman year of college, and unbelievably not only did my health not improve, it really began to slip.

With the addition of cafeteria food, my bowel movements became irregular. When I did go, it was accompanied with pain, mucus, blood, and chronic hemorrhoids. After my second year, a candida infection called Tinea Versicolor covered my skin, causing more embarrassment. My ability to concentrate and focus was seriously compromised, and the brain fog was especially thick and heavy. I was not doing well with my studies, even though deep inside I knew I was intelligent enough to be the best. I felt like a prisoner in my body.

The summer of 1999, desperate for relief from the continuous pain in my shoulder, I opted for shoulder surgery. The surgeon told me that my labrum completely ripped off and my rotator cuff was torn. Surgery was performed and he did the best he could, but was pessimistic about a full recovery. After the surgery I had a "frozen shoulder" despite going through a full course of physical therapy. Each time I moved my left arm, a creaking sound emanated through the room.

More surgeries followed. My tonsils were removed because of chronic infections. I was told further surgeries would be required on my left and even right shoulder. My left Achilles tendon snapped and rolled up my leg. Diagnosed with irritable bowel disease, I went through the indignity of several colonoscopies.

To say that my stress levels were immense would be an understatement. One night while studying, I ran my hand through my hair and a huge clump landed on the book I was reading and augmented my anxiety. Often the anxiety would not let up for weeks, or even months.

For years I battled a chronic cough and excess mucus in my lungs. Every morning I would wake up, cough for 15 minutes, and hack up globs of green mucus. I felt like garbage all the time. I was sure I had lung cancer, and I was scared. Despite the fact that my father was a physician, my mother was a nurse, and I was in pre-med, I found no answers.

I hadn't even lived a quarter of a century and all this was happening. When I felt I couldn't take it anymore, at my lowest and darkest moments, I decided to make a real change.

After consulting with my father, I decided to quit the pre-med program. My brother Brian influenced my decision to move to St. Louis and finish my B.S. degree in Human Biology. He was in chiropractic school and encouraged me to attend. I resisted because I thought chiropractors were quacks, but he convinced me to at least try. This was a momentous and difficult life decision because it meant that I was to break a five-generation tradition of becoming an M.D.

The drastic change of how chiropractors look at the body led me to a remarkable discovery that would not only save my life but become my passion. I slowly became aware of the principles that lead to health. This discovery fueled my passionate pursuit for learning and led me to read thousands of books, attend hundreds of seminars, and be treated by many great doctors in a search to find the secrets to unlocking health.

Through all this I gained a deep awareness and understanding of a paradigm of health called "The Cellular Theory of Health." The enormity of this concept led me to the works of renowned physicians and scientists like Hippocrates, George Goodheart, Francis Pottinger, Royal Lee, Claude Bernard, Weston A. Price, and Hans Selye, whose stories will be told further on. I realized that, since ancient times, successful physicians had adhered to the Cellular Theory and in doing so had healed what many of us believe are "incurable" illnesses such as cancer and heart disease.

By applying the knowledge I learned, I discovered the causes of my illness. I found that the nerve energy of my body had become diminished from several twists in my spine from the accident. I discovered that I had a frozen diaphragm and was not breathing completely, therefore my body had become overly acidic. Tests showed allergies to gluten and dairy, along with a leaky gut. I became aware that I was poisoning myself with processed foods, sugar, and other toxins from my diet. Simple tests showed I was deeply deficient in minerals and certain fats, that I was exercising improperly, and had adrenal exhaustion.

As soon as I applied the steps described in this book to my own health, my ability to self-heal exploded. The results were nothing short of amazing. I felt like I was experiencing a miracle. I fixed my chronic shoulder pain, and today I can lift both arms completely over my head with no restriction or pain. My flat feet healed. I no long wear braces in my shoes, and I frequently walk and run barefoot with no pain. It has been a decade since my last shoulder dislocation, despite a very active lifestyle that includes hunting, sailing, kayaking, and travel. My digestion normalized, my skin cleared up, and my energy returned. I described the new way I was feeling as "Whole Body Health."

The tests to reveal these problems are simple and inexpensive, and the solutions are mostly self-administered and can be done at home. The point of this book is to reveal all of this to you.

With a desire to help others to whole body health, I went on to receive a doctorate in chiropractic, learned the art of Applied Kinesiology, and became a nutritional expert. I built Whole Body Health Clinic in 2004, a multidisciplinary healing center.

At the clinic, we apply healing techniques described in this book. We use kinesiology, chiropractic, functional nutrition, physical therapy, oxygen therapy, laser Acupuncture, sound healing, whole food supplements, and diet to heal patients. Since opening, I have witnessed thousands of patients fully recover from their ailments. Many came to us as a last resort.

For the last 20 years, since I have become aware of the Cellular Theory, I have been working to find a universal healing formula that can help any condition. This book explains how the Cellular Theory dictates that we are the product of our environment. So to create a universal healing protocol, I synergistically combined health protocols that address each element (earth, air, water, fire). I found, to my great amazement, that when combined they exponentially multiply the benefits of each other, creating a power of healing for any condition.

By doing this I have discovered THE PATHWAY to beating disease. This is a monumental claim, but I know this works. It worked for me, and everyone I have applied it to gets better. If they're not past a tipping point, they completely heal.

This discovery inspired me to write this book to assist as many as I can to the joy of whole body health. Herein are contained vast amounts of information, gathered and condensed into simple and essential steps for healing. Though the instructions are easy to understand, to follow them requires commitment, discernment, and a strong purpose for healing.

Fortunately, you don't need to wear a white coat nor spend years pursuing a degree to understand this formula and its application.

Reading this book will be a rollercoaster of emotions, so hang on. You will at times feel inspired, at other times angry. You will laugh and have lots of a-ha moments. By the end of the ride, your paradigm of how you look at health and the world we live in will change.

In the first half of this book I lay out the philosophical basis of this formula and help you to understand the foundations from which it's built. I will examine the cellular theory of health and the history of its discovery; then contrast this with Western medicine, its beginnings, and the theory that drives it.

My goal is for you to use this book to connect the dots and simplify your path to achieve whole body health. Allow this book to be the signal through all the noise. Simply focus on the signal, follow it, and head toward Whole Body Health, letting nothing deter you.

I now believe that my life changed for the better on that fateful day when that car ran over me. It sure didn't seem like it at first, but the accident was a blessing and part of a bigger plan. I hope that blessing brings you healing.

2 - THE TRUTH

So are you ready to learn the story of how and why we got so sick and the simple solutions? Truth can sometimes be painful. Ignorance is bliss, or at least until you get sick. Waking up, seeing the chains and realizing that you need to make a change is difficult. The movie *The Matrix* put this concept forth quite well:

> *"It is the wool that has been pulled over your eyes to blind you from the truth... unfortunately, no one can be told what the matrix [truth] is, you have to see it for yourself. This is the last chance you have, after this there is no turning around. You take the blue pill you wake up in your bed and believe whatever you want to believe, you take the red pill and I show you how deep the rabbit hole goes...Remember, all I'm offering is the truth, nothing more. Follow me."*

The following pages pull the veil back and reveal the story of modern medicine and the simple solution to complete self-healing. Once you learn how to become your own physician and improve your health, you'll wonder why this information isn't taught in elementary school. You will become free from fad diets, prescription medicines, and the pain of being unhealthy.

If you're overweight, this book is for you. If you're in pain, always tired or depressed, this book is for you. If you can't use the restroom without great strain, don't cycle properly, lack libido, received a diagnosis, or simply want a more vibrant life, this book is for you.

This book does not address the medical treatment of any of these conditions; yet, in the end, it can solve them all. It will teach you how to harness the powerful

13

and innate healing properties of soil, air, water, and most importantly, your own body.

So, why are so many of us sick? When we get sick, why is it that our automated response is to take a drug? How many "blue" pills were force-fed down our throats to make us this way? How many drug commercials drilled our brains with easy "fixes," when deep down we already know the truth?

When we live unhealthy lives full of stress, and eat foods that have little nutritional value, inevitably we gain weight and get sick. Our automated response? Instead of considering lifestyle or nutrition, we go to an M.D. who prescribes drugs to suppress our symptoms.

Sad to say, doctor visits further the destruction of human health. The number one cause of death in this country is not car accidents, war, starvation nor disease.[1] It is iatrogenesis—which literally means "interference of medicine." Diseased people in various stages of meltdown are frequently made sicker by doctors through things like opioids, unnecessary surgeries, etc. Many of us accept their diagnosis and are led to believe that the only option to get better is patentable, expensive pharmaceuticals.

Recently, I saw a 35 year-old female patient who was extremely depressed, full of anxiety, riddled with poor digestion, and in constant pain. When I asked her about her history, she told me that she was diagnosed with bipolar disease, ovarian cysts, high cholesterol, and rheumatoid arthritis. All this at only 35!

With these diagnoses in hand, she was prescribed Effexor and Xanax for the emotional disease and had a hysterectomy for the cysts, which led to the prescription of synthetic estrogen. She was given laxatives for her slow bowel movements, cholesterol medication,

Prednisone for her arthritis and Nexium for her heartburn.

Her doctor was probably well-intentioned, but hopelessly compromised by a system designed around diagnosis and drugs. ~~The M.D. did not tell her that 90%~~ ~~of serotonin (the "feel-good hormone") is produced in~~ ~~the gut.~~ The M.D. also failed to acknowledge that the recommended antacids actually slow digestion, which results in more heartburn. Additionally, antacids block absorption of essential trace minerals and necessary vitamins, increasing her emotional issues.

How could an M.D., steeped in about 12 years of education, not see these obvious malfunctions? Was the M.D.'s solution to detoxify her liver, recommend a whole-food diet devoid of GMO grains and sugar, recommend plenty of sleep and rest, and heal her broken colon inexpensively with fermented foods and enzymes?

Not at all. Instead, the M.D.'s decision was to

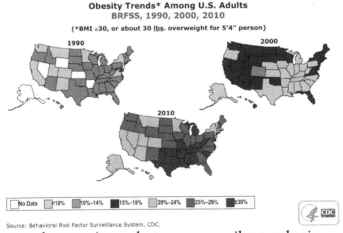

Obesity Trends* Among U.S. Adults
BRFSS, 1990, 2000, 2010
(*BMI ≥30, or about 30 lbs. overweight for 5'4" person)

No Data | <10% | 10%–14% | 15%–19% | 20%–24% | 25%–29% | ≥30%

Source: Behavioral Risk Factor Surveillance System, CDC.

remove her ovaries and uterus, prescribe synthetic hormones that are *proven* to cause cancer, prescribe addictive psychotropic medication to block her serotonin uptake, and give her a prescription antacid and laxative for life.

But really, her doctor is not fully culpable. Until now, this unfortunate woman, along with much of our population, did not know how to take responsibility for her own health.

Society essentially directs us to "not step out of line, go to work, and if you break down, the medical complex will give you a pill to fix it." We believe this because of brainwashing (advertisements), mis- and dis-information (government food pyramid anyone?), and corporate malfeasance (pharmaceutical companies work the cost of litigation from deaths and side-effects into their budgets).

The questions need to be asked.

Is heart disease caused by a lack of statin drugs? Is cancer caused by a lack of chemotherapy? Is osteoporosis caused by a lack of Fosomax? Is it possible that giant GMO companies like Monsanto, food companies like PepsiCo, insurance companies, pharmaceutical companies, medical schools, hospitals, and the FDA are all in bed together?

Why are 38% of us getting cancer[2] and 68% of us overweight[3]? The CDC says that diabetes is going to triple in the next 30 years[4] and cancer is the number one cause of death in children.[5]. How does this happen? Shouldn't we look at the root cause of this?

Is donating money to "charities" and research really the answer?

Is it possible that our food is ground zero for all these problems?

According to the University of Florida's research, the average young American male produced approximately 100 million sperm per milliliter of semen in 1929; in 1973 the average sperm count was 60 million/ml, in 1980 it was 20 million/ml, and it continues to drop.[6]

What in the world is happening?

A 1974 U.S. Senate investigation discovered that 2.4 million operations performed each year are unnecessary and kill approximately 12,000 people.[7] How many more is it today? Why hasn't the U.S. Senate conducted another investigation in the past four decades?

The CDC recognizes that 9 out of the top 10 causes of death can be attributed to diet and lifestyle issues. Yet, insurance doesn't pay for whole food supplements and lifestyle coaching. Why? Why isn't our Congressperson stumping on this topic on the campaign trail?

The only solutions and answers being offered to us by the medical complex are more research, more drugs and more healthcare. But is it working?

America spends 17.2% of our Gross Domestic Product (GDP) on health care, $3.2 trillion. No other country on Earth spends more than 10% of GDP on health care, yet in 2015 there are 45 countries with lower rates of infant mortality.[8] In its 2000 report, The World Health Organization ranked American healthcare 37th in overall health outcomes.[9] In an absurd attempt to make us healthier, on average, every man, woman, and child is prescribed around 13 drugs per year (and this doesn't count the over-the-counter drugs that people take on their own). Just 12 years ago, Americans were on average prescribed less than eight drugs per person, a 62 percent increase![10] Where does this increasing drug game end?

Why do we blindly accept medications from doctors, who are paid to prescribe them? ProPublica, a non-profit investigative journalism organization, researched how doctors are paid to prescribe medication and found that from August 2013 to December 2015 doctors received $6.25 billion in disclosed payments from pharmaceutical companies—and not all payments are reported.

How much are pharmaceutical companies really paying doctors to prescribe drugs?

The *New York Times* recently uncovered the fact that Pfizer admitted to paying $20 million in the last six months of 2009 alone to 4,500 doctors for "consultation" and to speak on their behalf (and this doesn't include payments to doctors outside of the U.S.).[11] Considering that there are about a million M.D.s in this country, the question begs to be answered: How much was paid to the remaining 995,500?

It's time that facts, science, and public demand challenge the status quo.

Money and power must not obviate scrutiny. If conventional health treatments do not stand up to honest, intense, and unadulterated inquiries, then logically, they must be abandoned until they can.

To continue to profit off other people's illnesses is psychopathic and destructive. This is your wake-up call. Awareness is the first step toward Whole Body Health.

How can we wake up? By seeking truth! The truth is that we can treat and heal our bodies naturally, inexpensively, and effectively and only then can we free ourselves. Only you can understand that your body has an innate healing system designed to cure you from anything. Darkness, like illness, can only by destroyed by letting in light. This book describes how to let the light in and build health, not how to fight the darkness and disease. So do you want to stay in the dark or do you want to know the truth? Do you want to take the blue pill or the red pill? Do you want to be fat, sick, and a statistic, or would you like to take action and heal yourself?

Have you answered the question? The choice is yours. If you take the red pill and continue to read, I will show you how deep the rabbit hole goes. *"Remember, all I'm offering is the truth, nothing more."*

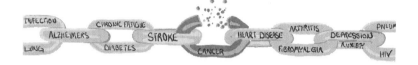

3 - THE BREAKING POINT

"The pattern of disease or injury that affects any group of people is never a matter of chance. It is invariably the expression of stresses and strains to which they are exposed, a response to everything in their environment and behavior."
—Calvin Wells, "Bones, Bodies, and Disease"

Two and a half millennia ago, Hippocrates became the first physician to put the concepts set forth in the following pages. He revealed the simple truth of human health and disease.

Hippocrates knew that naming diseases and treating them was next to useless. Instead, he understood the threshold that allowed disease to enter the body. He grasped the idea, then clearly conveyed it, that in order to bring the body to a state of homeostasis, the body's innate, natural healing abilities had to be ignited through natural processes. Once ignited, the body can heal itself.

Hippocrates was slow in administering drugs because he knew it made the work of a physician and the patient more difficult in the long run. The side effects increase stress in the body, ultimately causing unexpected new breakage along the chain of health, allowing illness to return.

Before Hippocrates, the pervasive healthcare belief was that disease was beyond anyone's control, and often a cruel curse of omnipotent and uncaring gods. He changed that way of thinking with the radical assertion that health depended on individual responsibility.

He went further to say that disease was the result of too much stress. The body can handle only so much until it falls out of ease. Once a threshold of stress is reached, the breaking point happens.

His solution to maintain and regain health was to address the stress points and remove the stimuli that are creating the disease in the first place. As basic as this may sound, it was a monumental moment for humanity and shook the paradigm of the day.

He was the first to state that diseases were caused by our environment. As a result, he came up with a simple system of diagnosing the root causes of disease and providing solutions for getting rid of them. He warned about the tipping point when living goes awry. He described it "as the point of imbalance in which illness triumphs and the patient succumbs to its effects"[12] and the power of healing diminishes.

He referred to this power of healing as "nature." In other words, nature is the body's innate power to heal and balance. He explained it can only do so below a specific stress point. He was the first to reveal the secrets of healing in writing, with statements such as "Let food by thy medicine and medicine be thy food," "Rest is of capital importance," and "Use only clean water or wine where used on wounds," which are self-evident today, but were not as clear to human civilization at that time.

Hippocrates taught that when you're stressed and your body begins to show signs of stress (i.e. fatigue, bad digestion, mood and hormonal swings, pain, cancer, diabetes, etc.), the solution was to eat good food, rest and change your environment (food, air, water, thoughts, etc.) to get back to wellness.

Yet somehow in modern day we have developed a healthcare system that cares nothing about our environment (food, air, water, etc.) We blame our afflictions on genetics and foreign infectious invaders, much like the ignorant ancients blamed their afflictions on angry gods. We have forgotten the simple truths that Hippocrates first spoke thousands of years ago. We have forgotten that our body is a temple and how we treat it determines everything about our lives.

Modern Studies and Research Prove Hippocrates' Theories Correct

Hippocrates' observations 2,500 years ago have been repeatedly proven. One modern study that stands out was outlined in a book by Dr. Walt Stoll entitled *Saving yourself from Disease-Care Crisis*. He tells a story about a study of stress, rats, and rabies.

In this study, rabies was injected into brains of rats to observe its effects. As expected, most of the rats contracted rabies and eventually died. However, some of the rats did *not* contract the rabies virus and stayed healthy.

The curious researchers further studied the surviving rats. For the second round of the experiment, they added a variety of stressors to the surviving rats, such as irregular feeding schedules, extremes of hot and cold temperatures, flashing lights, loud noises to disrupt sleep cycles, and other implements of rat torture.

Within a short time, all the remaining rats contracted rabies, and perished. What happened? The rats reached their threshold of stress *then* they broke. They withstood the first round of rabies injections because their healthy bodies were not overly stressed. The other rats went past the threshold that their bodies could handle. That's why they died in the first round of the study.

During the second round, the scientists ensured that the surviving rats reached their breaking point. They weakened their bodies with additional stressors. As a result, the rats' health reserves became depleted. Once their health "battery" drained, they succumbed to their weakest link of their health chain, which was the injected rabies virus floating around in their brains and blood. The virus triggered, because the rats' immunity broke and, unlike the first round, wasn't strong enough to repel it.

A scientist named Hans Selye proved this concept with modern studies. Known as "the father of stress research," Selye understood stress and its triggers and breaking points. He confirmed Hippocrates' observations with documented studies on stress and immunity conducted during the '50s and '60s in America. He identified three phases of stress. His research paved the path for the Whole Body Health formula by introducing a core concept of healing: Reduce and eliminate physiological stress and recover by adding in more things that support the body.

Chronic stress induces a civil war inside the body, and if you are constantly under stress, the casualty ends up being your health. When the body perceives stress either emotionally, physically, or chemically, it instigates a myriad of events to handle it.

Our bodies have developed this strong stress response as a requirement for survival. Evolutionarily speaking, when a stressor, such as a saber-toothed tiger or an invading enemy tribe showed up, our bodies required an immediate response. Anything short of extreme output from the body equated certain death. Over generations of natural selection, humans became hardwired for stress. An extreme stress response allowed us to preserve our lives. Without it, our ancestors would have died and we wouldn't be here.

However, modern life has developed an environment that has taken our stress responses to a whole new level. We have no rest. We are under constant bombardment of stressors, many of them invisible to the naked eye, such as toxins, pollutants, and work-related irritations. It never lets up. The result is an epidemic of disease sweeping modern life.

Selye found that there are three phases in stress breakdown from a healthy body to disease. How stressed are you? Keep reading and decide which phase of stress you are in.

3 Phases of Stress

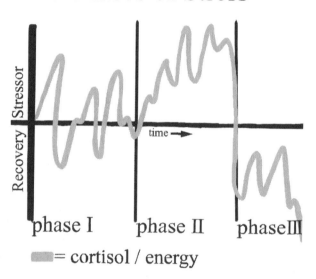

= cortisol / energy

THE SCIENCE OF STRESS

PHASE I—NORMAL RESPONSE AND RECOVERY

In phase I of stress response, our nervous system perceives a need for a response to a stressor. Our nervous system relays a message to the hypothalamus in the brain to produce and release a chemical called corticotrophin (CRH). CRH travels to the pituitary gland, which produces the adrenocorticotrophic hormone (ACTH). ACTH in turn goes to the adrenal glands, which produce a hormone called cortisol. Cortisol is the master stress hormone influencing every tissue in the body.

This system is referred to as the **HPA axis (hypothalamus, pituitary, adrenal axis).** It is, essentially, the processing system of stress response for the entire body. In other words, this is our "survival instinct."

Cortisol instigates a cascade of effects. It immediately releases stored sugars from our liver for quick energy to the muscles. It diverts blood flow from our internal organs to our muscles, so they engage in rapid "fight or flight" response. The body shuts down digestion, quickens the heart rate, and shortens the breath.

An example of this could be seen if a terrorist ran into your room right now firing a weapon. In response, you would immediately have a charge of energy to fight him or jump out the window. Either action could save your life, and this is normal, healthy, and essential. It evolutionarily ensured the survival of the human race.

Once stress goes away, the body recovers to a state of balance. Rest helps the body recuperate quickly and fully, and prepare to handle the next inevitable stressful event that life throws our way. Ideally, we cycle between periods of stress and recovery, always returning to a state of homeostasis and health.

In this phase, people don't feel ongoing daily stress. They respond normally to stressful situations and then they recover. In other words, they're healthy.

PHASE II—CHRONIC STRESS

Compared to our evolutionary ancestors, modern living overwhelms us with constant daily stressors, never giving us a chance to recover.

Let's examine a typical modern day. Many of us start the day off with a blaring alarm after a restless sleep. After our morning routine, which may be harried depending on how many times we hit the snooze button, we consume a high-starch breakfast, a pot of coffee, and jump in a vehicle to fight traffic.

We spend 8 to 12 hours in a work environment that is a minefield of numerous stressors. Then we fight traffic again to get home and numb our stressful day with more stressors like TV and alcohol.

The next day it's the same. It feels like we're in a race all day long, every day. Indeed, this is the American 'rat race.' Hopefully, nobody's injecting rabies into your brains.

Life exposes us to obvious stressors, like a fight with our loved ones or rush hour traffic. However, modern living takes our constant stress exposure to a whole new level, accumulating it at an alarming rate. Measurable, yet invisible, stressors such as EMF (electromagnetic frequencies), chemically spiked food and water, and air pollution are ever-present.

Our body has no choice. It responds the same way our ancestors did when they crossed paths with a vicious saber-toothed tiger. All 'modern stressors' initiate the HPA axis to respond continuously, without rest.

Hormone levels increase and glands enlarge. We live in a constant state of fight or flight, continuously battling invisible tigers and terrorists.

We repeat this daily stress routine, often without ever getting a significant break. In phase II, our body rises to meet the stress effectively, but we are entering a dangerous state of being.

A lot of us actually feel good in phase II. Life's hard, but we somehow manage to keep up, maybe even excel. This phase can last many years, until we feel ourselves coming to the end stages of phase II. We notice symptoms of constant fatigue, pain, or some other ailment. So we try to compensate with caffeine, sugar, medications, and a host of other stimulants, essentially whipping our bodies like a jockey does his exhausted horse in a last desperate sprint towards the finish line.

Then one inevitable day, something finally breaks.

PHASE III—BREAKING POINT

The reality is that our endocrine system can only handle a finite amount of stress. The body can only take so much before it collapses. Our health plummets as a result of the continuous stress response. Our battery of wellbeing is drained, and only the residue of toxicity accumulates.

Visible negative changes in our body appear. Seemingly overnight, we look and feel old. Joints hurt. Libido disappears. Exhaustion, inflammation, weight gain, and brain fog settle in. The brain malfunctions, making even simple tasks difficult.

Our stress response diverts vital energy to the heart. Stomach acid and enzyme production nearly halts, leading to a downward spiral of poor digestion and lessening nutrient absorption.

We reach a crisis phase. Drained of energy, we magnetize disease. Bacteria, viruses and parasites lick their chops as the weakened body becomes an easy target for their malfeasance.

The body has reached its max allostatic stress load. Disease names, doctor visits and endless medications roll in. Disease overcomes.

This is not theory. Thanks to Hans Selye's research, it is documented scientific fact.

Allostatic Stress—The accumulation of Bad Stress in the body

Some stress, however, is actually good for the body. This is the basis of the concept of hormesis. With hormesis, you gain after an initial pain. Take exercise, for example.[13] Without stress, nothing on earth could function.

Just enough of the right type of stress actually stimulates healing.

Author Nassim Nicholas Taleb coined the term 'Anti-Fragile,' a concept that precisely defines and illustrates hormesis.

It is an essential concept that must be understood to regain and maintain health, and achieve peak living. Things gain with disorder and chaos (stress). Anti-Fragile means that something must actually break in order to get better. Countless examples throughout history—in nature, societies, and individuals demonstrate the benefit of a specific, small, or therapeutic dose of anti-fragility.

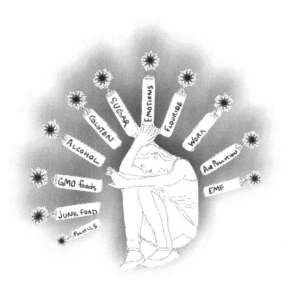

Cumulative allostatic (The medical term for accumulation of stress in the body) stress, on the other hand, is **chronic stress with no benefit.** Substances like sugar and alcohol have no benefit. Neither does chlorine, fluoride, mercury, asbestos, cyanide, or lead. Nor do the 80,000 other currently known toxins in our environment, nor the 2,000 new ones introduced each year.

Drinking a sugary soda, breathing polluted air, and showering in chlorinated water all encourage failure somewhere along the chain of health. Allostatic stress load contributes to breakdown, all the time, without exception. It results in dysregulation of multiple physiological systems such as weight gain around the belly, depression, high blood pressure, cancer, etc.

When physiological systems break down, the cellular terrain of the body changes for the worse, reaches a tipping point, and disease quickly ensues. Modern medicine futilely attempts to restore health by diagnosing which link is under the most tension. Then it tries to suppress the symptoms with drugs and invasive techniques. This serves only to transfer the strain to another link in the health chain, actually moving one closer to the final breaking point, thus accomplishing the exact opposite of curing illness. Modern medicine, more often than not, adds to the allostatic stress load.

For example—*and this happened to me*—repressing acne with a chemical cream manufactured by a pharmaceutical company might repress the acne today without addressing the root of the problem, which is poor nutrition and toxicity. Continued poor nutritional intake along with the side effects of the medicated cream results in worse symptoms down the line; perhaps a candida infection, liver damage, or a colon malfunction...and so it goes, unless the allostatic stress load is reduced by eliminating toxins such as the acne medication itself, and introducing nutritionally dense foods into the diet.

Modern life's stressors are lesser an ultimate danger (we're not fighting saber-toothed tigers anymore), but those stressors are relentless and non-stop. Also, modern day stressors have radically increased in the last 150 years or so. A 1987 study showed that the average person in America is exposed to more than 1,000 times the stressors per person per day than people just 100 years ago.[14] How much more have we added in the last 30 years?

This is the most insidious threat to overall wellbeing since the dawn of man. From an evolutionary standpoint, we are incapable of dealing with it. Pick up a copy of any recent medical journal, and it's replete with studies of soaring obesity, diabetes, heart disease, and cancer rates.

So what do we do?

4 - Life is about making choices

"Wherever the art of medicine is loved, there is also a love of humanity." —Hippocrates

Life is about making choices. We choose where to live, whom to love, and what to eat. We consciously make these choices and know we have to live with the outcomes. What most of us don't realize, and therefore never choose, is which paradigm of health we want to follow when we become ill. Many don't realize there are two competing theories of the causes of health and illness.

The current healthcare model engineered for society is based on the germ and genetic theories of disease. This states that health is mostly outside of our control. Germs we catch determine which infectious diseases we get, and genetics determine which non-infectious diseases we're likely to experience.

When we get sick, we go to a doctor who names the germ or genetic disease we're experiencing, then uses drugs, surgery, or procedures to try to suppress or manage the disease process. Most of us are quite familiar with this theory.

The opposing theory is known as the Cellular and Epigenetic theories of disease. This basically states that all disease is created by too much stress and to heal we must reduce, and if possible, eliminate stress in our environment. Eliminating and reducing emotional, chemical, and structural stressors will result in health. In other terms, your body's natural defenses are strengthened by reducing stress and nourishing the body.

My father's favorite poem is Robert Frost's, "Two Roads." He recited it often to me, *"Two roads diverge in a yellow wood...I took the one less traveled by, and that has made all the difference..."*

When it comes to your health, you cannot choose both roads. We're either building up the body or tearing it down.

Think of it like this: When the stressors occur, like the terrorist running into the room with a gun, you can try to fight the terrorist or you can flee, but it's hard to do both. When your body becomes sick, you can attempt to drive the disease from the body with medications or procedures. While this may work, it always increases your stress load. A different option is to build up your body's natural defenses by reducing your stress and nourishing the body —it's counterproductive and ineffective to do both.

Before you can choose your path, it's important that you understand the history, theory, and dreams of medicine and contrast that with the theories behind the Cellular Theory of Health. Then make your choice.

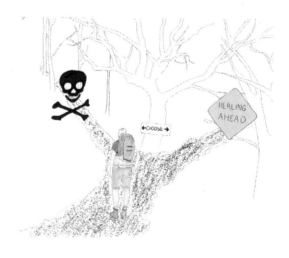

Choose wisely:

____**Paradigm I: The Cellular and Epigenetic Theory of Health**

vs.

____**Paradigm II: The Germ & Genetic Theory of Disease**

OPTION 1: The Cellular and Epigenetic Theory of Health

"One of the biggest tragedies of human civilization is the precedence of chemical therapy over nutrition. It's the substitution of artificial therapy over nature, of poisons over food, in which we feed people poison in trying to correct the reactions of starvation" —Dr. Royal Lee

It comes down to this: There are two opposing forces in the universe. Organizing intelligence that heals vs. random disorganizing and chaotic forces behind disease.

The effective application of the Whole Body Health formula relies on a thorough understanding of a little-known theory of health called "The Cellular and Epigenetic Theory of Health" that harnesses the creative and healing forces of organized intelligence.

This concept, though simple, may seem hard to wrap your head around at first, as it's a completely different way of thinking about health and disease. However, as Albert Einstein brilliantly said, "We can't solve problems by using the same kind of thinking we used when we created them."

The power behind holistic healing that Hippocrates named "The Power of Nature" has also been referred to as "Innate," "Universal Intelligence," the "Tao," and the 'Power of Creation.' It is organized energy that powers an organism to greater intelligence, resulting in self-healing. The power that made the body heals the body.

Organized intelligence permeates nature. Regardless of whether you believe in creation or evolution, the unifying theme underlying both is organization. A foundational principle in physics is that energy tends to randomize more and more as the durations of time continue. Yet, somehow we find ourselves in a harmonic galaxy on an organized planet with an incredibly complex nervous system that senses and witnesses it all.

Examples of organized intelligence exist throughout the natural world. Look around a garden and contemplate it for a moment. Realizing the organizing power of nature leaves us in awe. Growing plants convert light from a star 93 million miles away into oxygen and energy. A food-chain hierarchy of insects and animals with organized digestive systems breathe that oxygen and feed on those plants and each other. Those animals defecate, die, and eventually go back into the soil, giving plants the necessary bio-matter to continue growing. The beautiful symmetry and intelligence of nature allows all life on earth to appropriately function with grace.

We see this organization extend into outer space, where a cosmos is ordered so perfectly we create dependable calendars and timepieces based on orbits of galactic bodies. The earth spins, tilts, and rotates in a symmetrical organized manner around the sun. Meanwhile, the solar system journeys around the Milky Way and the Milky Way moves through the universe with a sense of purpose we are just beginning to observe and barely understand, though we grasp its heavenly grandeur and gaze at it all in open-mouthed wonder. It's as though all life through all galaxies has all been orchestrated into a beautifully choreographed dance. Who is the conductor?

Humanity marvels at its own technological breakthroughs. "They are marvelous," we say, "because they are inspired by and mimic nature." However, technology represents but a fraction of nature's intelligence. Radar systems use sonar to track and find objects in the skies and oceans, though not nearly as effectively as a bat. Planes employ the same principle of lift that birds naturally adhere to without jet fuel and engines. Cameras seek to replicate what human vision sees, but the photograph is a faded snapshot, lacking the vibrancy of that moment that an eyeball captures.

The most amazing example of all, in my opinion, is the intelligence of the human cell. Each cell is able, through a system of neurological and hormonal connections to signal surrounding cells, activate DNA, selectively take up nutrients, and like a small nuclear reactor convert calories into energy. Simultaneously, it repairs itself, reproduces, and through a complex set of equations, auto-destroys at the end of its useful life. The technology that it would take to replicate even one human cell is unfathomable. Yet, 100 trillion comprise your body to work divinely in seamless unity when healthy.

Somehow, even though it permeates nature, many humans, and most doctors, believe that organized intelligence is reserved for our own minds and imagination. Instead, limited technological thinking produces cures using man-made chemicals. Ultimate universal intelligence is ignored, even though it is obviously within and all around. It has been said that all the computers in the world put together do not have the computing ability of one human-being's nervous system.

Life is a mystery. All we really know is that for the brief moment we're here we are exposed to constant duality. It permeates all of nature. We witness light and darkness, positive thinking and negative, lift vs gravity, birth and death, disease and health. What so many physicians have witnessed and attempted to name in their own words is the indescribable power of nature termed "Universal Intelligence," which runs the body's ability to autocorrect imbalances. What this book is really about is how to harness that power and emphatically turn it loose in your life. By increasing the organizing energy of the body and reducing the chaotic stress, your ability to heal magnifies. Even if you don't believe a word you've read, you have to marvel how a wound mends itself before your very eyes. This is not random. It's a powerful healing act of organizing universal intelligence.

This energy is everything. Without it: No cellular function, no metabolism, no life. With it: Abundant creation and healing. This was the belief of Hippocrates, Claude Bernard, D.D. Palmer and thousands of other great healers throughout history.

In the mid-1800's, it all changed with Louis Pasteur. His new theory laid the foundation for the modern medical industry. His "germ theory" of health stated that we are surrounded by 'bad' bacteria and exposure is the cause of disease.

However, Claude Bernard and Antoine Béchamp, two French scientists who were contemporaries of Pasteur, developed the competing paradigm of "Cellular Health Theory," which they originally named "The Cellular Theory of Disease." This theory states that infectious organisms take root once universal intelligence is lost and the cellular environment is weakened.

When the body loses EASE, then DIS-EASE emerges. They found through their work that germs, parasites, bacteria, and viruses are *attracted* to dead and dying tissue as stressors build up and cellular function drops.

Disease occurs not because destructive bacteria overpowers a healthy cell but because disease is attracted to a weak, poorly functioning one like flies to a pile of smelly manure.

Furthermore, the theory holds that a healthy cell's immune system repels unhealthy organisms and disease, much like a Jedi warrior uses the Force to throw around stormtroopers.

Another way of saying this is that we don't get exposed to bad bacteria, then get sick and then need medication. First we get weakened from stressors (sugar, toxins, medication, lack of nutrition, etc.), then we get sick and finally bad bacteria arrive.

This theory was further proven by Nobel Prize winner Otto Warburg's research when he measured the charge of healthy human cells. He used the apt metaphor of a battery to describe cell and body function. He discovered that the battery's charge is determined by measuring the production of ATP (adenosine triphosphate). ATP is literally the substance of energy produced by the cells. If the human cell is fully charged and recharging, ATP production is plentiful. As cellular charge decreases, so does ATP.

Our bodies become acidic as stress runs down our cellular batteries. The more acidity in the body, the higher likelihood of disease occurs.

Healthy human cells range between 100-70 millivolts (MV). When our cells become stressed and drop below 70 MV, bacteria and fungus appear. When cell voltage drains to below 40 MV, chronic illness begins and viruses appear. Below 40 MV - cancer, heart disease, and death quickly and assuredly ensue.

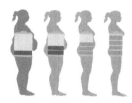

To reverse this life force, cells must recharge. Alkalinity in the tissues must be restored for healthy function.

Measuring cellular charge and salivary pH is an effective method for determining levels of health. I perform it on every patient that comes into my office. Once the cellular charge and pH is known, progress is easily monitored by measuring how much the cells recharge during the healing protocol.

Application of 'The Cellular Theory' is easy. Chemical medication is unnecessary. Instead, build a strong and healthy cell that retains a high cellular charge. The stronger and healthier the cell, the less likely that disease will occur. A healthy cell also recharges its battery efficiently and quickly. In medicine, this is called a 'holistic' or 'functional' approach to healing.

The ultimate premise of this theory is that only *the body can heal itself,* and it can only happen if you're providing it the tool that it needs to do so. It is the basic tenet for Whole Body Health. Once you comprehend it, you can answer questions such as, "How can I build stronger cells?" and "How can I increase the flow of universal intelligence throughout my body?"

The other half of this paradigm features the Epigenetic Theory, which basically states that your environment determines whether genetic diseases express themselves.

The concept is simple. Let's say you have a genetic marker for a lymphatic disease. It might "switch on," developing lymph node disease, if your environment is a high stress job, in a polluted and busy city, drinking fluoridated/chlorinated tap water, with heavy industries pumping toxins into the air, while being bombarded by EMF and radio waves, light pollution, noise pollution, extreme weather and crime.

If you live in a healthy environment, however, the genetic marker won't trigger the lymph node disease. This healthy environment could be a place where you eat real food and avoid exposure to endless toxins. You may even do things in this place that you love such as fishing, stargazing, and salsa dancing with your friendly neighbors on Friday night.

Living in an environment that promotes homeostasis will not trigger genetic markers for disease, though it does run the risk of triggering perpetual smiling! Studies show that our environment is 10 times more influential than our genetics at birth in determining our health.[15]

So why would Angelina Jolie remove her breasts, despite the fact she had no cancer? Because she has the genetic marker that signals a possibility of breast cancer? I recently read that she had a full hysterectomy too. Essentially, she's castrating and mutilating her body because of fear from a test indicating that she has a likelihood of contracting cancer, but only if she leads a stressed life.

Who is her doctor? Why is her doctor not telling her the truth that it's the terrain matters? Angelina, if you are reading this, please, do not mutilate your beautiful body. Please! Instead, buy an estate away from it all. Go there to relax and live life fully (even if it's not with Brad Pitt), and I would be happy to be your personal physician. Seriously, I'm not kidding. I'd take that job in a heartbeat.

Since the time of Hippocrates, this truth has gone from theory to documented scientific fact. The evidence is overwhelming. The health of the cellular terrain is everything! It doesn't matter if there are E. Coli bacteria in your gut, which there is right now by the way, or you have latent tuberculosis in your lungs, which many of us currently do. It only matters if you make your body too weak to restrain its spread.

Currently, and sadly, the truth of Cellular Theory is violently opposed by those in power. German philosopher Arthur Schopenhauer described three stages truth passes through: Ridicule, violent opposition, and finally acceptance.

Stage one: Truth is ridiculed. An idea seems silly at the time because no one's ever heard or thought of it, (i.e., "There is no stinkin' way the earth is round you idiot.")

Stage two: Truth is violently opposed—Generally by the power structure in place. As it gains ground, people whose power and hierarchy is threatened by the new paradigm react to it violently and persecute the perceived threat. People are starved, maimed, hanged, shot, crucified. Many times, there is great sacrifice, blood flows for truth, and this is why it is rare to see it publicly. Truth requires strength, bravery, and leadership, (i.e., "You say you are the way, the truth and the life? Crucify Him boyzzz!")

Stage three: The truth is accepted as self-evident, (i.e., "Of course the Earth is round! I knew that all along. What do you think I am, an idiot?")

Since the time of Pasteur, the "Cellular Theory of Health" has been in the second stage of truth. Sadly, documented history reveals persecution of doctors and scientists to keep this simple truth of health from spreading.

The good news is that it's impossible to suppress the truth forever. Fortunately, we crossed the threshold into a period of awakening. This is self-evident by the fact that more and more people are demanding real health care and real food. Many people are seeking to clean up our environment instead of tearing it down. We are entering into the third stage of truth.

If you choose to follow "Cellular and Epigenetic Theory" and the way of Whole Body Health, the vibrational healing frequency of your cells will intensify. As you become aware of your environmental stressors and choose to add more positivity into your life, your body will harmonize with the mind to create new thoughts and patterns of joy. Realization of a better existence will emerge and healing will occur. Once you become a fully aware warrior, always seeking positivity and avoiding negativity, there is no limit to your life. Disease is only the expression that fills the void when health is lost.[16]

OPTION II: The Germ & Genetic Theory of Disease

At the end of times the merchants of the world will deceive the nations through their Pharmacia. - Rev 18:23

Western medicine subscribes to the Germ and Genetic Theory of Disease.

The first aspect of this theory basically states that bacteria (or viruses or some other destructive microorganism) are the cause of disease. Therefore, the way to health is to destroy the invading bacteria and preemptively build defenses against them. Thus, the industry of "pharmacia" manufactures antibiotics, vaccines, and pills based on chemicals to suppress and eliminate "bad" microorganisms.

Louis Pasteur believed that if you could eradicate bacteria, health would be restored and maintained. He recommended processes of sterilization for food that are his namesake: pasteurization, which to this day is the corporate food standard. In theory, if bacteria are killed in the food, there is no, or at least a lesser chance of disease. He was also the first to suggest vaccinations in an attempt to create artificial immunity.

The second aspect of the theory is that genetics determine which non-infectious disease to which we'll likely succumb. For example, if you have a family history of leukemia, the likelihood of developing it is higher, no matter what your health protocol. Therefore, the weak genetic link for leukemia must be preemptively treated or attacked to prevent the disease from happening. Since the human genome project completed its mapping over 20 years ago, the promise of bio-engineered cures has still not been fulfilled. Yet today, this belief still holds firmly. Billions of research dollars and thousands of lab reports later, we're still waiting with bated breath.

This path is called "allopathic medicine." This is the current dominant model of healthcare that's been in place for nearly 100 years.

"Allopathic medicine" continues to use radical surgeries, toxic medication, damaging radiation and other extreme invasive techniques in a failed attempt to aggressively drive disease from the body.

On paper, The Germ Theory approach seems solid. However, it's ineffective for long-term whole body health. The reason is simple. Unless the cellular environment is healthy, bacteria, and disease always come back stronger and better equipped to handle medicine's eradication efforts.

In medicine, this is referred to as the "bi-phasic" effect.

Cancer treated with chemo often results in further cancer, because even though radiation destroys the cancerous cells, the integrity of healthy cells surrounding the cancer are also severely compromised, thus curtailing their ability to resist the very cancer that chemo is trying to destroy. Bacteria treated with antibiotics return as super bacteria. Allergy medication stops your response to an allergen, giving the illusion of ridding it. But in actuality it drives it deeper into the body forcing an even stronger immune response down the road, requiring more medicine to suppress it again, and the cycle repeats until it breaks you.

Surgery is the same. Perform one spinal operation and the likelihood of needing a second doubles; get a second one and it doubles again.

There is no end to the game of allopathic suppression techniques.

The "bi-phasic effect" is common throughout all of allopathic medicine, directly contributing to worsening disease conditions.

This is quite apparent in the prescription patterns of all pharmaceuticals. Negative side effects are inherent with every prescription. Once a patient starts one medication, a new symptom or disease pops up, so doctors prescribe another drug to cover up the side effects of the first. This is known as prescription cascading and turns into a condition known as Polypharmacy.

The only tool available to combat disease for most doctors is drugs. Many feel they must do *something* for the patient sitting expectantly in front of them, so they prescribe almost every time someone walks in the door. As a result, doctors get caught up in the pharmaceutical industry's reward system, discouraging medical professionals to recommend a safer path to healing.

An easy drug fix quickly cascades to dozens of prescribed medications. Most people agree to it because insurance pays for it and a trusted doctor recommends it. The Journal of American Medical Association has found that 50% of prescriptions are prescribed improperly, leading to devastating side-effects. Even "properly" prescribed medications result in 1 in 5 people developing serious side effects that account for 120,000 deaths annually.[17]

In America today, on average, every man, woman, and child is prescribed 13 medications per year. Additionally, they are almost never taken off previously prescribed drugs. In 2011, American doctors wrote 4.02 billion prescriptions.[18] That's a lot of drugs sold! A drug dealer should be so lucky!

Modern medicine's dream was never to create health, but rather to sell as many drugs and procedures as possible—from prenatal care, right up to death in an effort to manage disease.

An example of this corporate greed is the story of Martin Shkreli, who made headlines for hiking the price of a drug called Daraprim from $13.50 per pill to $750. His response to the backlash and criticism to this obvious greed? "My shareholders expect me to make the most profit, that's the ugly and dirty truth."[19] Thank you for taking those exact words out of my mouth, Mr. Shkreli. At least he's being honest about it. They are in the disease management business. It's lucrative. Profits trump healing.

This allopathic approach is utterly failing. The leading cause of death in America is 'iatrogenics,' which literally means "death by medicine," Around 800,000 people die each year directly from poor doctoring.[20]

Over the next decade, scientists predict that iatrogenic deaths will total about 7.8 million, more than all the casualties from all the wars fought by the U.S. throughout its entire history, a death rate equivalent to that caused by six jumbo jets falling out of the sky every day.[21]

According to an independently funded and peer reviewed report by the Nutrition Institute of America, the path of modern medicine and its application of "The Germ Theory of Disease" and "Genetic Theory" has resulted in a diseased state. Many people have become hapless victims, unable to cope with their own symptoms, reliant on a medical and pharmaceutical system that employs extreme techniques with devastating side-effects. Each time a person takes a drug, allostatic stress increases, moving them closer to the ultimate breaking point.

It's terribly sad how many of us are sick. I know what it feels like to be sick, to be a recipient of countless doctor visits, drug prescriptions, procedures and diagnoses. I know what it's like to be told I have to live with a condition for life. It's devastating. It's a nightmare.

We must wake up to the hard truth that medicine's allopathic approach doesn't work at preventing or curing disease. The germ theory of disease is wrong and drugs don't cure. The best it can do is "manage" the condition, and even this is debatable.

Allopathic medicine is easily criticized when it comes to healthcare. But to be fair, where allopathic medicine shines is with emergency lifesaving care. This is why allopathic medicine is referred to as "heroic medicine." Emergency medicine and antibiotics have saved my life and members of my family.

Antibiotics too have a place in medicine, but are vastly overused, and now their age of efficacy is coming to an end.

I am proud to say that my father was a brilliant emergency room physician for over 20 years and he saved thousands of lives. But even he agrees that emergency care, antibiotics, and drugs should be reserved only for life stabilizing conditions. The continued application of "emergency care" as healthcare denigrates quality of living.

"Emergency only" care has actually been documented to be the most effective form of medical care. How do we know this? Data collected during the rare times that doctors go on strike.

The Social Science and Medicine Journal conducted a review of doctor strikes and the resulting health impact on their surrounding area. The study analyzed five different doctor strikes between 1976 and 2003 with periods ranging from 9 days to 17 weeks. In every single one of these historical events, the mortality rate either remained the same or decreased. There was no increase in deaths![22]

The most remarkable example of this was in Los Angeles County in 1976. Doctors went on strike to protest malpractice insurance premiums that were gouging their incomes. They provided emergency care during this five week strike, but all routine office visits were denied. The result? At the beginning of the strike: 21 deaths per 100,000. At the end of the strike? 13 deaths per 100,000, a 40% decrease in deaths![23]

Empirical observation dictates the following medical care model: No heroic medical measures of drugs or surgery are ever necessary, short of an immediately life threatening situation and only for a short time. All drugs for non-life-threatening situations should be stopped as soon as feasible. Emergency medicine, the aforementioned heroic medicine, is the only requirement for healthcare.

If this were law, hundreds of thousands of lives would be saved each year.

"But I must see my doctor routinely," you might protest, "to maintain my health and make sure there is nothing wrong." Are you sure about that? The British Medical Journal recently posted a meta-analysis of all studies analyzing routine medical visits. The conclusion? "General medical checkups in adults do not decrease morbidity and mortality from disease."[24] Not my words...

Currently, pharmaceutical companies justify their position by calling their approach "evidence based." Other forms of healthcare are dismissed based solely on *their* subjective evidence.

Medicine, even today, is not based on scientific assertions. Only 11% of recommendations by doctors for heart disease are considered scientifically valid. The Journal of the American Medical Association (JAMA) states: "Heart disease is amongst the most studied illness in all of medicine, yet just 11% of ... 2,700 recommendations approved by cardiologists for treating heart patients are supported by high-quality scientific testing...The proportion of recommendations for which there is no conclusive evidence is also growing. These findings highlight the necessity to improve the process of writing guidelines and to expand the evidence-base from which clinical practice guidelines are derived."[25]

Yet our country continues to spend over $100 billion every year on heart surgeries alone.[26] Medicare spent $46 billion on blood pressure medication in 2011[27]. $29 billion was raked in by cholesterol medication[28] despite no valid studies proving their long-term benefit.

According to WebMD, the cost of cardiovascular disease in the U.S. was about $444 billion.[29] If only 11% of 444 billion is supported by high-quality scientific testing, perhaps the rest can be abandoned.

Dr. Richard Horton, editor-in-chief of the Lancet, states that at least half of scientific literature published today is simply untrue.[30] Dr. Marcia Angell, former editor and chief of the New England Journal of Medicine said, "The pharmaceutical industry likes to depict itself as a research-based industry, as the source of innovative drugs. Nothing could be further from the truth."[31] John Ioannidis, epidemiologist at Stanford University of Medicine, wrote an article called "Why Most Published Research Findings Are False."[32] I could go on forever.

The fact is medicine and government should be kept separate, just like religion and government, to maintain a truly free society. The for-profit pharmaceutical system continuously manipulates the government to serve its economic interests by maintaining it serves the "public good" while massively enriching itself.

I'm reminded of what E. Richard Brown wrote:

"The crisis in today's health care system is deeply rooted in the interwoven history of modern medicine and corporate capitalism. The major groups and forces that shaped the medical system sowed the seeds of the crisis we now face. The medical profession and other medical interest groups each tried to make medicine serve their own narrow economic and social interests. Foundations and other corporate class institutions insisted that medicine serve the needs of (their) corporate capitalist society. The dialectic of their common efforts and their clashes, and the economic and political forces set in motion by their actions,

shaped the system as it grew. Out of this history emerged a medical system that poorly serves society's health needs."[33]

The very paradigm on which medicine is based is faulty. For all the money spent, treatments given, and studies performed, the cure to disease (heart, cancer, etc.) will never be reached using "the Germ and Genetic Theory" of health.

Going after disease rarely works, but the opposite path of pursuing health always helps. Let me repeat Mother Teresa's quote, "I will never attend an anti-war rally; if you have a peace rally, invite me."[34] She understood.

If you are unhealthy and want to get better, why would you want to walk into a building that says "Cancer Center" in big letters on it? Wouldn't you rather walk into a building called "Whole Body Health?"

Please don't misunderstand. I am not criticizing scientists, doctors, or researchers, but only the corporate greed that has created the system. Many of these people are good souls who truly want to heal humanity, but are hampered and even imprisoned by this business model.

Ironically, the same scientists and doctors that created the problem will be necessary to right many of its wrongs. My hope is that the medical and pharmaceutical industry develops courage to step out of a dysfunctional system and actively participate in a solution that is better for all.

Want to know how we ended up at this juncture in healthcare? Want to know how this modern lie started? Want to know who's responsible for building this atrocious business model?

Keep reading, and learn about the villain who started it.

5 - ROCKEFELLER MEDICINE

"Competition is Sin"—John D. Rockefeller

The history of our current medical system is a dark and interesting drama of greedy people manipulating governments and society to implement a drug-based medical system.

Filled with intrigue, villainous personalities, persecution, and heroic characters, most of it is beyond the scope of this book. However, it's important to understand a brief history of allopathic medicine in this country in order to make an informed decision on which path of healthcare to choose.

The story of how it all began is really the story of one person: John D. Rockefeller. This story is not my opinion or a parable. This is how it happened according to historic documentation.

In an endless pursuit of money, Rockefeller sought to monopolize medicine, as he had the oil industry, and started the Rockefeller Institute of Medical Research in 1901. The institute was designed to be America's first biomedical drug-based institute and, like France's Pasteur Institute, was based on Pasteur's theories.[35] The institute's director of laboratories was a man named Simon Flexner.[36] With powerful capitalistic motives, they wove a dark plan to dominate the healthcare business in America and then the rest of the globe.

Rockefeller sought to build a medical empire capitalizing on allopathic medicine, despite the fact that he himself flatly refused allopathic medicine. In fact, his own physician was a homeopathic practitioner named Dr. Hamilton Fisk Biggar.[37]

Rockefeller worked closely with the powerful philanthropic organization, The Carnegie Foundation, because he needed a layer of deniability between his interests and the healthcare system he was rigging.[38] He influenced the Carnegie Foundation in 1908 to hire Simon Flexner's brother, Abraham. Abraham was brought onto the research staff, and his duty was to present a report to U.S. Congress. The report's subject was about the state of medical research and schools in America. The little known but incredibly impactful piece was called *The Flexner Report*. It's available on Amazon if you want to read it.

Abraham Flexner was a preacher in Massachusetts when he was hired. He was not a physician, scientist, or medical educator. He never set foot in a medical school before evaluating them for his report. In fact, his only schooling was a two-year degree in the *classics*, making him completely unqualified to decide which types of medicine were scientific and valid and which were not.[39] Regardless, his views were submitted to Congress in 1910.

Flexner adhered to the germ theory of medicine and believed anything other than this approach was tantamount to quackery. The Flexner report disseminated falsehoods under the guise of science and ruthlessly slandered all other methods of healing that competed with pharmaceutical medicine. Time-honored traditions such as homeopathy, nutrition, manipulation of the body by osteopaths and chiropractors, electromagnetic therapy, acupuncture, and others were persecuted and deemed "non-medical and unscientific."[40]

After submitting his report to Congress, he no longer needed to keep a layer of deniability between him and Rockefeller. In 1912 he was hired to the Rockefeller

Foundation's General Education Board and in 1917 became its secretary.

After the Flexner Report was published, the number of medical and health colleges in America decreased from 189 to 31.[41] A carrot and stick approach helped accomplish this.

The carrot was a big one: Tax-free donations totaling to about $600 million (inflation adjusted) to medical colleges that "fit in" with his agenda[42] with the requirement that he could put his people on the boards of the schools.

The stick came in multiple forms. First, licensure and accreditation was restricted to only the colleges that met the Flexner Report's requirements.

Second, the American Medical Association (AMA) and FDA were used as their henchmen. In 1910, the same year that the Flexner report was published, the AMA published *Essentials of an Acceptable Medical College* (Report of the Council, 1910), which echoed similar criteria for medical education and a disdain for "non-conventional" medical study.[43]

The AMA's head of Council on Medical Education traveled with Abraham Flexner to evaluate medical schools for the report. Medical sociologist Paul Starr wrote in his Pulitzer Prize-winning book: "The AMA Council became a national accrediting agency for medical schools, as an increasing number of states adopted its judgments of unacceptable institutions." Further, he noted, "Even though no legislative body ever set it up...the AMA Council on Medical Education's decisions came to have the force of law."[44] It's important to note that the AMA is not a government agency. It is a private, for-profit organization, flush with money.

Third, they set up an attack group called, and I'm not making this up, "The Propaganda Department." The Propaganda Department's sole purpose was to run baseless smear campaigns. Dr. Fishbein, MD wrote in his autobiography, "In 1913...the AMA working with Rockefeller went on a strong offensive by establishing the 'Propaganda Department,' which was specifically dedicated to attacking any and all 'unconventional' medical treatments and anyone (MD or not) who practiced them."[45]

The AMA referred to any health practitioner as "quacks" if they were not part of their organization. They ruthlessly and doggedly persecuted anyone they perceived as competition to their business model. Medical students of the day were taught not to associate with anyone who did not follow the allopathic path of medicine as they were 'quacks and inferior.'

During this bleak period in medical history, any university not using the methods condoned by this new business model was censured. Most eventually shut down. Many holistic doctors were jailed for "practicing medicine without a license," and over the following decades, holistic methods and ancient healing techniques went underground. Sadly, some were lost entirely.

After changing the course of medical and health education in America, Flexner, with funding from the Rockefeller Foundation, was sent to Europe and according to author Thomas Bonner, came to be known "nearly as well in Europe as in America." Bonner went on to say, "Flexner exerted a decisive influence on the course of medical training and left an enduring mark on some of the nation's most renowned schools of medicine."[46] After Rockefeller controlled the legislative bodies and schools in both America and Europe, he went on to stack the FDA with his own men, ensuring rubber stamp approval for pharmaceuticals and a barrier for entry to all other forms of healthcare. This ensured that pharmaceutical companies supplied the entire nation's medicine. This began the medical system we know today. Medicine was monopolized and corporatized, into an extremely well oiled money-making machine.

Society's choice for healthcare was reduced to one: Allopathic Medicine. All other forms of healthcare were persecuted and many were eliminated. Any survivors had to go underground or practice outside the new system. The population was not made aware of any other choices of healthcare. Society was engineered to believe the illusion that Allopathic Medicine was the only form of healthcare.

Despite this obvious coup of the medical industry manipulated by Rockefeller, the Yale Journal of Biology and Medicine in 2011 wrote "The Flexner Report of 1910 transformed the nature and process of medical education in America with a resulting elimination of proprietary schools and the establishment of the biomedical model as the gold standard of medical training."[47] These 'proprietary schools' discarded centuries of healing wisdom, taught by some of the greatest physicians in American history. The cruelty of this destruction is unfathomable when the great loss of knowledge and teachers is considered. I guess the old saying is true, "History is written by those who have killed heroes."

Dr. Benjamin Rush, a signer of the Declaration of Independence, said, "Unless we put medical freedom into the Constitution, the time will come when medicine will organize itself into an undercover dictatorship. To restrict the art of healing to doctors and deny equal privileges to others will constitute the Bastille of medical science. All such laws are un-American and despotic." His words have never rung more true.

6 - THE SHIFT TO THE SUGAR AGE

"The earth does not belong to us. We belong to the earth. Whatever befalls the earth befalls the sons and daughters of the earth. We did not weave the web of life, we are merely strands in it. Whatever we do to the web we do to ourselves."—Chief Seattle

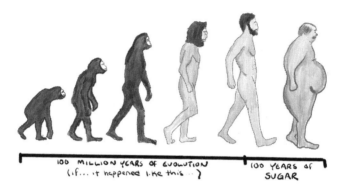

100 MILLION YEARS OF EVOLUTION
(if.... it happened like this ...)

100 YEARS of
SUGAR

Because of a shift away from the cellular theory toward chemical therapy, our health has shifted. There is a palpable shift of the human experience of life. It can be pinpointed to the beginnings of the twentieth century. Our way of living and what is important to us is incongruent with our ancestors' way of life and collateral casualties of this shift are visible.

In this chapter you'll learn, despite stats that say the opposite, why we're actually the most unhealthy human culture in history, what created this shift, how corporate and government intervention in our food and healthcare system are solidifying and profiting off this shift, and finally the simple solution to it all.

According to the Centers for Disease Control (CDC) we're living longer than ever and the increasing average life, which is currently 78 years of age, is the proof. It is argued that this increase in lifespan is due to advancements in technology and medicine.

I beg to differ. Not on the fact that our average life expectancy is at 78, but that it's due to advancements in "modern medicine." This is a well-designed lie. As Benjamin Disraeli said, *"Lies, damned lies, and statistics."* Let's investigate.

On December 18, 2003, Reuters ran a story on the impact of AIDS in Africa. The reporter wrote, "A baby girl born now in Japan could expect to live 85 years, while one born in Sierra Leone probably would not survive beyond 36." The point of this article was to highlight how medicine and technology result in a longer life. The average person is not dying at 36 in Sierra Leone. In actuality, the high infant mortality and crime rates, along with a lack of sanitation, is pulling down the number. The average person who avoids these calamities in Sierra Leone will most likely live the same length as one living in Japan.

Let's do an analysis of history and an examination of the CDC's claims. The encyclopedia of life states that the average life expectancy in prehistoric times was probably about 25-30 years, and in medieval Europe it "improved" to 36 years. Conditions back then were harsh with no central air, smartphones, or Starbucks, making life particularly brutal.

Sure, the life of a caveman was probably short. Brutal death occurred more often than not by woolly mammoth trampling, saber-toothed tiger hunts gone awry, starvation, or freezing.

Medieval European life's brutality was a bit more refined. Painful skewering by a lance during jousts, walking through rat infested, crap-filled, crowded streets, and fighting in useless feudal wars for some duke made for many possibilities of ending a man's life sooner than later. Women didn't fare well either, with constant witch hunts and whatnot.

150 years ago in America, the Civil War raged, and to this day the casualty count from it is the highest of all of America's wars. Surgery at the time was usually conducted with a bottle of booze, not to pour on the wound for disinfection, but to be drunk by the patient as anesthesia. Quite advanced, I must say.

All kidding aside, there are running threads of commonality during these periods of human history that affected true "average" life expectancy.

One thread is that childhood mortality was atrocious. Death at birth was common, both for the baby and the mother. Until about 150 years ago, many children died before they made it to 5 years of age. If they made it that far, the next 13 years of life was fraught with potential ways to die from infections and accidents.

There was little understanding of sterility for treating wounds and injuries. Infections were common because there was no central sewage system. People often lived in cramped conditions and threw garbage and human waste in streets. There was no hand washing. In effect, we existed in an unhealthy environment that served as a breeding ground for dangerous bacteria, not healthy human bodies.

If people made it past 18 years of age and survived war, our ancestors generally lived to 80 or beyond.

We are fed the conventional narrative that humans live longer because of 'miraculous' medical advances and technology. It's tempting to congratulate ourselves for developing a progressive society whose knowledge surpasses previous "primitive" generations. The false historical impression given is that by the time we turned 40 in Medieval Europe, we were old, unable to move around without a cane, or on our death beds. Nothing could be further from the truth.

When we talk about "average life expectancy," we are saying "life expectancy at birth." This is described as the length of life the average human can expect to enjoy in any given country, unless some freak accident should befall them.

Life expectancy at birth has probably never changed. Hand washing and plumbers did far more to enhance average life expectancy than doctors. Hand washing at first wasn't even accepted by the medical community. Ignaz Semmelweis, now described as the "savior of mothers," found that the incidence of puerperal fever at childbirth could be dramatically reduced with hand washing by medical caregivers. In 1847, at the time of his discovery, hospitals' birth wards had a rate of mortality three times that of midwife wards.[48] He published his findings in his book *Etiology, Concept and Prophylaxis of Childbed Fever.* For some unfathomable reason, his views conflicted with the established scientific community. He was committed to an asylum and beaten to death 14 days after his arrival.

I have a good friend, a retired plumber, who proudly states as often as he can, "The health of the nation depends on plumbers, and we don't get nearly as much money as doctors." Though plumbers are expensive, they are worth it. The proliferation of modern sewage systems and household plumbing coincided with the advent of vaccines and antibiotics, yet it barely gets the credit it deserves for improving average life expectancy. These medical outsiders have done more to improve overall human health than our modern medical system today, whose charges are comparatively and considerably outrageous. Gallbladder removal for $15,000? Seriously?

Life is like a candle. Your life explodes into light as you're thrust into this world at birth and that light of life continues to glow for all of your days without fading. That's where the song, "This little light of mine" came from. We all know how it goes: "...this little light of mine, I'm going to let it shine, let it shine, let it shine, let it shine..." When your time is over, the life light flickers briefly, and we die quickly.

We are witnessing something different, however. The average person now spends years at the end of their life needing assistance. After a prolonged period of dimming, their light slowly goes out.

Our life expectancy at birth has probably not increased, and the quality of our health in these modern times has declined precipitously, especially as we age. Generations past were quite active even into their advanced years. There was no such thing as a nursing home. Home healthcare, if it was necessary, was provided by the children.

Today, you have a 68% chance of disability if you're 65 years or older.[49] In other words, for 68% of us over 65, life is going to be hard. We're not going to enjoy a quality life of freedom. You may not be able to wipe your own butt, take an unassisted bath, or drive a car.

According to projections from the U.S. Census Bureau, the number of disabled elderly will double by 2050.[50] Imagine that, a country half-full of disabled people.

The tipping point of any society is when there is not enough healthy people to care for the unhealthy ones. How close are we to this tipping point?

Diseases such as obesity, diabetes, and Alzheimer's are skyrocketing. One in three people can expect dementia for the last years of their life. Cavemen could not afford these diseases. It would've significantly interfered with their ability to evade the aforementioned woolly mammoth trampling.

Many lives today degenerate into listless countdowns to death in old people prisons that we call nursing homes. People often abandoned by their families, cared for by corporations, staffed by exhausted and emotionally hardened nurses, and kept "alive" with chemical medications.

What happened? Why is our quality of life (happy, usable years) shortening, though the length of our life remains the same? What is failing us? Is the business of long-term care and prescription medication really the answer?

What created this shift?

Let's start with food and take a broad look at the evolution of diet. What follows is a general description. We can go deep down this rabbit hole, but for now we'll summarize 99.99% of our evolutionary diet in a basic overarching manner.

The food we ate was whole and unadulterated meat, vegetables, fruits, fish, nuts, insects, etc. The only processing, if any, was cooking, drying and curing, pickling or fermentation. Much of our food was consumed raw. During our hunting and gathering phase, which by the way is about 99.9% of our evolutionary existence, humans ate mostly a balanced meal of meat and vegetables. Sweet foods such as fruit and honey were the Holy Grail, and consumed seasonally, or when available as a rare treat. Edible vegetation grew wild in thick, deep fertile soil profoundly enriched with trace minerals, probiotic bacteria, and nutrients in a beautifully complex ecosystem provided by nature and her universal intelligence.

With the advent of agriculture, we'll say about 8,000-10,000 years ago, grains and money came into the picture, as did the first sign of cavities in human skulls, as did merciless resource extraction. It's all downhill from there as far as Earth's and humanity's overall health is concerned.

Mass sugar plantations and cultivation developed about 500 or so years ago, correlating with the rise of more cavities. Nonetheless, at this period, sugar was still considered a rich person's food. The poorer you were the less you could afford sugar for much of recorded history.

People happily settled for honey and fruit seasonally; it was plenty of sugar, and each year they looked forward to it, maybe even celebrated it with harvest festivals. Rare ailments linked to its overconsumption were confined to nobility. If you saw a fat man hobbling on a cane in diabetic pain, it was most likely a duke who at tea time could afford to gorge himself on lumps and crumpets. Instead of thinking the guy was unhealthy, people might have said, "Man, he's rich!"

Only kings and nobility could afford to be fat. Obesity was a "disease of the rich" and ostensibly a social status. In fact, some believe that Marie Antoinette contributed to the violence of the French Revolution when during a famine she uttered the now famous words, "If they don't have bread, let them eat cake." "Cake?" the starving commoner most likely uttered, "They have cake? Let's cut their heads off and steal it!"

The peasantry of centuries past ate bone broths. They made stew out of "leftover" animal carcasses, throwing in hearty vegetables like cabbage, carrots, beets, leafy dark greens, and whatever vegetation/herbs that were edible. Cooked slowly, each bowl was savored with gratitude.

As it turns out, they were preparing and eating nutrient dense foods. It was the poor who ate "cheap" foods, which of course turned out to be today's "health" foods.

The dietary divide between rich and poor quickly shrunk during the expansion of America. Massive industrial and shipping operations dramatically increased accessibility and consumption of sugar, especially in the past 100-150 years.

In the 16th century, four pounds of sugar was the average per capita consumption in Europe. As people became addicted to sugar, the demand for it skyrocketed. To fuel this demand, the New World was exploited. Native cultures were ruthlessly enslaved to run plantations. Modern society's new addiction was sugar, and it needed more.

By 1880 sugar consumption jumped over 700% to 29 pounds average per capita. Today in America the average person consumes at least 150 pounds per year, with children often consuming the most. That's a 3,750% increase in less than 500 years.[51]

This is where the shift happened. All of a sudden rich people's food became affordable to the rest of us.

Processed foods and chemicals became the norm, and organically grown meat and produce became the expensive rich person food. Historians will look back on this shift, as they have the Bronze Age, and surely they will call it, *The Sugar Age* or perhaps, *The Corporate Food and Healthcare Age*.

The Beginning of THE SUGAR-AGE & Government and Corporate Interference in Our Food

At the turn of the 20th century, the U.S. government witnessed the beginnings of the shift. Alarmed at the developing health crisis, regulations were enacted and bureaus were established to try to hold back the tide of disease washing over the nation. The sugar and chemically processed-food-lobby formed in response.

Dr. Harvey Wiley, the highly respected original head of the FDA (then known as the Bureau of Chemistry), wrote the book *Foods and Their Adulteration*. His first course of action was to enact the "Pure Food and Drug Act" into law in 1906. This law attempted to control the American food supply's purity. It outlawed usage of preserving chemicals, saccharin, bleached flour, and other denatured food products. Dr. Wiley knew these substances were literally poisonous. They lacked fiber, enzymes, vitamins, and mineral content, and were directly linked to all levels of digestive problems. High fructose corn syrup was not around at the time, otherwise it surely would've made the list.

Six years later Dr. Wiley lost the good fight. A powerful refined food industry lobby formed. Their relentless attacks finally achieved their desired effect. His coerced resignation was accepted in 1912. He was replaced by a pawn of the industrial food industry.[52]

The modern *sugar age* had officially begun. It was off to the races for the processed food industry. Profits were handsome. However, the disease it spread turned out to be fat and ugly.

Dr. Royal Lee said it best, "When a food manufacturer sells you a denatured product, he is shortening your life for his profit."

In a stunning turnaround from trying to protect citizens, the government's next stage in the development of the the sugar age was to actually reward people who create industrialized food with subsidies, thus encouraging more industrialized food.

Sugar and Processed Food Subsidies

What is a subsidy? Simply put, subsidies are government handouts of money to privately owned businesses and corporations. Subsidies are a fancy way to say "corporate welfare" or "farm income stabilization." They are a hefty tax burden as the U.S. spends more than $20 billion per year in subsidies.[53]

Subsidy programs started in the 1920s, but really took hold during the Great Depression. The U.S. isn't the only country that subsidizes its farmers, however. Subsidization in the U.S. impacts international trade affairs the most, causing all sorts of havoc in global commodities markets, and contributes to global poverty and starvation.[54] Cheap, subsidized food commodities are dumped into Third World countries. Local farmers simply can't compete with the cheap crops, and they are driven out of business. Third World countries in turn become reliant on these dumps, and borrow money to buy. As wealth is funneled out of the country, insurmountable debt contributes to poverty and destabilization of the countries' infrastructures. Starvation ensues in a twofold manner. Firstly, the subsidized GMO crops are nutritionally inferior. Secondly, local farms and businesses are shut down, and the loss of income and jobs makes even the cheapest food unaffordable.

The original intent of subsidies, though convoluted, was honorable. It was the government's attempt to control manipulation of commodities markets and supplement farmers' incomes. At the time it was implemented, 25% of the country lived on about six million small rural family farms . Today, 157,000 mega agribusinesses represent 72% of total farm sales.[55] From 2003 to 2005 the biggest 1% of these mega-corporate farms received 17% of all federal subsidies (roughly $2.14 billion).[56]

Somehow, subsidies have been perverted from a system of income supplementation for family farms to a mono-cropped nightmare of mega-business cashing in on taxpayer money. Thanks to subsidies, the sugar age blossomed.

Corn is, by far, the most highly subsidized agricultural commodity. Cotton, wheat, and soybeans round out the next three on the list.[57] Subsidized corn is used primarily for the manufacture of industrial and unhealthy food products, one of the worst of course being high fructose corn syrup (HFCS). HFCS is ubiquitous in modern processed foods.

Have you ever wondered why a hamburger, large fries, and soda "value meal" is around $5, yet the same food from an organic market is three to six times as much? Have you ever wondered how this is possible? If you ever tried to grow these foods yourself, you'd recognize that the water, soil, and human energy input required for even just potato cultivation is massive.

The ranch, pasture, feed, water, fencing, and human stewardship required to grow cattle for your burger is cost-prohibitive, and virtually impossible for one person to accomplish. So, how can a meal like this be only $5? The only way a restaurant can sell you a "value meal" is when the food in that meal is subsidized, thus encouraging its consumption.

To make matters worse, up to 40% of Americans receive some form of government food assistance, which is used to buy what is perceived to be the most affordable food available. This purchasing judgment usually results in nutritionally useless, highly processed calories, pumped out by an industrialized food system awash in subsidies.

Many people who received government assistance recognize this is not an ideal way to feed themselves, but are faced with a poverty of choice and need to fill their kids' bellies. So they settle for processed foods. Many have no choice as they live in a "food desert" in inner cities where no real food can be found or is grown.

Wouldn't it be better to subsidize healthy foods? How do you think health in America would change if a fast food "value meal" was $30 while an organic salad was $3?

The final nail in the coffin—Government sponsored health

In America, under our current healthcare system, the sicker the patient becomes, and the more testing and procedures they require, the richer the doctor gets.

This is exactly opposite from the way healthcare worked in ancient China where the physician was compensated by the patients as long as they were healthy. If the patient lost their health, the doctor lost their income until they helped them regain health. What a concept! Many doctors today making in excess of half a million dollars a year would drop to below minimum wage under this approach.

Our system is further destroyed by the patient who does not directly pay for, and therefore care, how many tests or procedures are done. I have had patients say to me, "do as many tests or procedures as you want as long as my insurance pays." This same patient when asked to quit eating fast food flatly refuses as this requires active participation and sacrifice from them. "Can you just give me more insulin?" the diabetic often asks.

Once people become ill from the food industry, they go to doctors who don't change the foods that are making them ill. How can you possible stop someone from dying from ingestion of poison if you don't take them off the poison?

The final straw in the person's health is when they go to a hospital. I was absolutely mortified recently when my mother-in-law got tongue cancer. I was astonished that the hospital fed her nutritionally empty and sugar fortified foods. Before chemotherapy and radiation, and at the end of each meal, they would offer ice cream. A hospital giving ice cream to a person who has cancer, potentially caused by ice cream, is tantamount to medical malpractice. She got a $300,000 bill for the chemo and ice cream that Medicare happily paid.

The current medical/government complex has created a society of individuals that do not seek all options of healthcare. In essence, the marketing of this system of insurance, medicare, and pharmaceuticals presents the illusion that this is the only choice. Furthermore, the illusion continues when people have a co-pay of only $50 monthly for $4,000 of medications. If someone was recommended gallbladder surgery, but they had to pay $15,000 for it out of their pocket, do you think they would opt for it? Or do you think they would search hard for an alternative that is inexpensive and actually effective in restoring their gallbladder function? If they had to pay for it out of pocket, do you think anyone would opt for these tests and medications? Without skin in the game, people won't try.

As radical as it may sound, the abolishment of health insurance (other than emergency care) would immediately impact society's overall health for the better. As long as doctors, pharmaceutical companies, and hospitals (and therefore legislators that are paid off by them) benefit from providing only "sick care" to the population, the more sick we will become. Our current medical is a system *proven* to cause more death and illness. Pharmaceutical companies, insurance companies, hospitals, the processed food industry, and of course Rockefeller and his family, are rewarded and further enriched by it.

Massive, collective symptoms of disease are the direct end-result of our profit-driven corpo-government system. As long as profits grow, we won't see true change. Sorry, Obama...and Trump.

The government shakes hands under the table with these corporations and does not issue legislation that truly protects the people. Then the government actually pays large agribusinesses to produce unhealthy processed foods, then subsidizes consumers to buy these crappy foods. People eat this toxic food, inevitably illness follows, and their only option for healthcare becomes government subsidized drug care. People are never shown any other option. The Physicians Committee for Responsible Medicine states that 63% of subsidies in the USA are causing enormous costs and burdens to the health and productivity of Americans.[58]

So why does this sugar age continue?

Why don't we subsidize organic healthy produce and stop subsidizing junk food? Why don't we subsidize only doctors who improve and maintain people's health?

Why? I'll tell you why. Lobbyists!

The corporate food industry spent an estimated $539,000 in 2008 for every daily session of Congress[59] and they're dwarfed by the pharmaceutical and insurance industries, which spent $400 million in 2015.[60]

I'm not saying anything revelatory here: the U.S. Congress and the health of humanity is for sale. This statement doesn't come as a shock to most Americans, who routinely give their federal legislators dismal approval ratings.

The real question is, how do we save ourselves from this corporate sick care system?

American soul food is a great example.

Captured and forcibly transported as slaves, people from the African continent have been disproportionately disadvantaged in American society. The impoverished black community of the past couple of centuries relished collards and greens cooked in broths and lard. Meat was treasured, and every single possible part of the animal was efficiently used, including organ meats. Fishing was a great source of protein, and all fish parts were used and cooked. Though not considered a delicacy as they are today, this community creatively manifested opulent feasts with ribs.

The result was that the poorest segment of American society, who endured atrocities of awful hatred, grew stronger because nutrition fueled their courage. Their diet was nearly perfect. High in fats and good proteins, and plenty of veggies cooked with it, or eaten raw.

The tragedy is that today's soul food is poisoned with sugar and other chemicals from the corporate food industry. The deplorable obesity, diabetes, poverty and crime rate in America is substantially higher amongst this demographic. Today's generation of African-Americans, along with the rest of the population, face their most dire challenge yet: the government subsidized, corporate agriculture, industrial food and health complex.

The words of Martin Luther King Jr. ring true to this day, "The time is always right, to do what's right."

Are you ready to step out of this disease system and free yourself?

70

7 - SOLUTIONS TO THE SUGAR AGE

"You have more control over your body than you think- you can control, manage, or completely avoid 60-70% of known chronic conditions with physical fitness, healthy nutrition, and mental balance." —Samir Becic

So, what's the solution? How do we free ourselves from the bondage of illness?

Those who are sick have always wanted to understand what secret sauce the healthy subscribe to. Ponce de Leone famously explored the new world for the fountain of youth. I searched when I was sick. You may be searching right now.

Despite globalization, there are still pockets of people living in balance with the earth and still maintaining excellent health. These regions are called "blue zones." A blue zone is a demographic/geographic area where exceptional health exists with longevity. Recently, Dan Buettner wrote a book about "blue zones" and their common characteristics. Some of the blue zones of the world include Okinawa (Japan), Nicoya (Costa Rica), Icaria (Greece) and Loma Linda (California).

To be among this elite group of people is the goal of life. Songs celebrate the blessing of a happy, healthy and long life. "To your health," is always the toast I give! This age-old search for this elite formula of an exceptional life continues today. What makes some of us better, more robust, happier and healthier than others? What elixir is the fountain of youth? What creates health and what do healthy people look like?

It is known and documented that the healthiest people on earth have wide symmetrical faces, straight teeth, clear skin, bright eyes, and good skeletal posture. Physicians routinely document these characteristics as signs of health when evaluating patients. When I was a young man looking for a wife I definitely looked for these things in a partner. We are inspired by and attracted to beauty, because we instinctively know it translates to fertility. Like rapper Sir Mix-A-Lot famously said, "I like big butts and I cannot lie...shake that healthy butt." Sorry, couldn't resist.

When settlers came to America, the first thing they noticed was that the native population was beautiful. They had good teeth, wide symmetrical faces, and surprising physical abilities—to shake those healthy butts. Why do you think John Smith fell in love with Pocahontas? It wasn't her money or language skills, I can tell you that.

The most common characteristic that all cultures have associated with beauty is symmetry of the face. Science defines this symmetry and measures the ideal ratio of the face as 1.62, based on Fibonacci's golden ratio. Dentists and plastic surgeons improve beauty by aligning a person's face closer to the magic 1.62 ratio. By the way, nobody is perfect, but my wife is pretty close!

95 years ago in Cleveland, Ohio an accomplished dentist asked these same questions. His name was Weston A. Price DDS. Looking day in and day out at his patients' teeth, he saw a dramatic rise in cavities, gum disease, crowding of the teeth and a narrowing of the shape of people's heads and palates. He noticed a pattern of disease.

These signs of failing health concerned him because he saw them spreading through all levels of society. In his seminal book "Nutrition and Physical Degeneration," he documents the decline of healthy characteristics in modern American society. Dr. Price called these dysfunctions (dental disease, mental disease, heart disease, diabetes, cancer, obesity, and inflammatory pain conditions) the "displacing diseases of modern commerce." Poor teeth and gums are a direct manifestation of poor health. As a dentist, Dr. Price was keenly aware of this. In his book, Dr. Price quotes Harvard physician Earnest Hooten, who stated:

"I firmly believe that the health of humanity is at stake, and that unless steps are taken to discover preventatives of tooth infection and correctives of dental deformation, the course of human evolution will lead downward to extinction. The facts that we must face are, in brief, that human teeth and the human mouth have become, possibly under the influence of civilization, the foci of infections that undermine the entire bodily health of the species and that degenerative tendencies in evolution have manifested themselves in modern man to such an extent that our jaws are too small for the teeth which are supposed to accommodate, and that, as a consequence, these teeth erupt so irregularly that their fundamental efficiency is often entirely or nearly destroyed."

Dr. Price, in an effort to understand the increasing American disease state, explored the world in search of the answers. He talked his wife Florence into a journey that would take them through 14 countries and five continents. We are the beneficiaries of that journey, as he documented the results in his book.

His travels covered both modern and isolated people. They included the Swiss, the Gaels, the Eskimos, the Indians in the far North and West, the Polynesians of the Southern Pacific, the Aborigines of Australia along with the Maori tribes of New Zealand.

73

Understanding the implication of this important experiment is inspiring. This observational study, this meta-analysis, on the scale Weston A Price performed can never be performed again because there are now few places on the globe with societies untouched by the diseases of modern commerce. Products like Coke-a-Cola, phytochemical fertilizers, and genetically modified food permeate every corner of the globe. Even if there were such an experiment today, most of his observations could never again be performed. We are in the midst of the grand human experiment.

During his travels, he encountered some civilizations that consumed mostly red meat, some that consumed no red meat. Some that ate extremely high amounts of saturated fat while others had low amounts. Some ate seafood while others had none. Some that had access to fresh fruits and vegetables and some that had no access. Some were near the ocean in tropical destinations and others were in the Arctic Circle. Yet despite these differences, he was able to document what made healthy cultures similar.

His point of entry into their health was teeth and gums, width of faces and dental palates. Upon arriving at a new village or island he would sit down with the leaders and ask permission to examine the face and teeth of the people that lived there. What he found was the healthiest teeth he had ever seen, despite the fact that most never heard of toothpaste, fluorinated water or dental floss. In fact, the first isolated people he visited, a Swiss village, had a green slime covering their teeth. But beneath this slime were perfectly healthy teeth without cavities. He found only 1 in every 100 teeth contained a cavity. A whopping 30x lower incidence of cavities than in his practice in Cleveland.

In his searches, he found the thread that held all of these healthy cultures together. In doing so, he rediscovered Hippocrates' formula for good human health. He observed that as soon as the people departed from their traditional way of living and separated from living in symmetry with the earth and were ingesting or were exposed to the displacing foods, water, and air of modern commerce, they quickly lost whole body health regardless of where they were on the planet. He found that there is really only one disease on Earth, the diseases of modern commerce and human greed. Sadly he documented the final demise of the few remaining vibrant cultures as the sugar age engulfed the entire planet.

Through it all, like a final life-line being thrown to a drowning population, he was able to document how these people lived, giving us a way out should we choose to follow. The principles he documented that led to Whole Body Health were reaffirmed by Dan Buettner in the study of the blue zones and cemented by my own observations and travels. It can all be summed up like this: **What we eat and the terrain on which we live mold us into who and what we are.**

"And when you want something, all the universe conspires in helping you achieve it." —Paulo Cohello "The Alchemist"

So what are the solutions? As we're collectively waking up to the bad decisions our leaders and moneyed interests have subjected us to, we must take responsibility for how we live if we hope to shift from the sugar age and Rockefeller medicine back to Whole Body Health. While it can seem overwhelming, the solution is simple.

It starts with you and your belief in yourself and the desire to invest in your own wellbeing. Gandhi said, "Be the change you want to see in the world." The first step is to quit buying subsidized processed foods. All of it, right now! Secondly, don't fall prey to the lies of an easy pharmaceutical solution to the illnesses caused by these foods.

As we heal ourselves, we must choose where we put our continued support. Where and how are we voting with our money? The only way that this sick system continues to propagate itself is through a blind consumerist economy. Without our dollars, it flounders and flails like a mythological beast slain by a hero. It's an incredibly powerful and effective vote for true change that evolves into a new system that cares for our planet and aligns us towards healing.

As more of us vote with our dollars, organic humanely raised food and real healthcare will spread throughout the world. Every time a restaurant or store goes "organic" or a "natural" healthcare clinic pops up, there is a ripple effect throughout the entire industry and the entire world. This is the only way real change ever occurs, because enough of us demand it. You can change the world by simply choosing to support what's right. Like Dr. King said, "the time is always right" and the time is right now!

The solution to it all was theorized by Hippocrates, documented by Weston Price, and fixed in my own mind by reading thousands of studies and books and personally giving over 200,000 patient treatments.

So here it is in its entirety. The pathway to Whole Body Health can be accomplished in 10 easy steps. Get ready, you are about to embark on the journey of your life and awaken to a new world.

1) We must activate the power of the mind when it comes to healing. This has been called "placebo" and is said to be the most powerful tool in medicine. By aligning our thoughts with healing, we will take a major first step toward its attainment.

76

2) We must eat *no* refined, processed, or denatured foods. All foods should be taken directly from the Earth without modifying or changing them.

3) We must seek to increase the nutrient and mineral density of food we consume by selecting only organic fruits and vegetables and wild- and pasture-raised meats.

4) We must seek to increase the enzyme and probiotic content of food and therefore our digestive capacity and metabolic processes. If our digestive system is already damaged or insufficient, then supplements must be taken.

5) We must improve our detoxification abilities to keep up with modern-day toxins.

6) We must turn our bodies into fat burning machines and fuel them by consuming healthy fats that are balanced in Omega 3 and Omega 6 and high in fat-soluble vitamins.

7) We must move much more each day than modern day life requires.

8) We must have clean oxygen-rich air to breathe.

9) We must have chemical free, structured, and alive water to drink.

10) We must increase the flow of universal intelligence through the body by using the Earth's most powerful medicines to scorch out the remainder of disease.

Hopefully the previous chapters about health, stress, the history and theory of medicine, and the cellular theory of health have prepared you, like fertile soil, to receive the seed of healing. The second half of the book is the manual describing specifically how to heal yourself. Remember though, the path is narrow and you must follow the formula exactly if you want results.

8 - INTRODUCTION TO THE MANUAL

OK, we're ready to begin our journey to Whole Body Health! It's imperative that you grasp the philosophy behind healing as painted in the first few chapters. The cellular theory of health states that we are a result of our terrain and the elements that surround us. If we surround ourselves with excess chemical, physical and emotional stressors, we will become sick. Conversely, healing requires us to synchronize our bodies and our minds with the elements of nature to promote what Hippocrates called "the power of nature."

The four elements of nature are Earth, Air, Water, and Fire. Negative stresses from the elements tear down our cells while positive inputs build them up. For the purpose of this manual I have broken down the steps of healing as to how they relate with the elements. Knowing how to control your elements is the way of the Whole Body Health and the art of healthy living.

There are many, many cures out there that have the potential to strengthen your cellular environment. While it's impossible to discuss them all, this book outlines the most important. The formula laid out in the following pages is sufficient for most people to heal themselves completely. Each element will list what actions should be removed and which should be added in great detail.

MIND:
REMOVE: Negative Thinking and Curses
ADD IN: A power statement of healing and finding your purpose for healing.

EARTH:
REMOVE: Sugar, Carbohydrates, and Processed
Foods Completely
ADD IN: Organic Food, Minerals, and Digestive
Support

AIR:
REMOVE: Inactivity and excessive CO_2
ADD IN: Indoor plants (or move to nature),
Diaphragm Stretches, Deep Breathing, and Aerobic
Exercise

WATER:
REMOVE: Fluorinated, Chlorinated, DEAD
WATER
ADD IN: Clean, Structured, ALIVE Water

FIRE:
REMOVE: Medications
ADD IN: Increased Sun Exposure, Chiropractic,
and if necessary, Cannabis.

Follow this program until health is achieved. For the
first three weeks of this program attempt to follow this
book to the letter, starting at the beginning. Many will
be happy with their progress after three weeks, some
will need to be perfect for months before health is fully
achieved, and everyone will need to change their habits
if they want to maintain health.
Before starting this program, some simple methods
of determining overall health should be performed. Seek
to get each of these tests into the healthy range before
quitting the program or experimenting with cheating.
These tests are listed below and described in detail
throughout the book. They should serve as the markers
of your progress.

You'll need some inexpensive equipment like a blood pressure cuff, pH strips, liquid potassium iodine (also known as Lugol's solution), and blood work. The cost of all of the equipment is less than one visit to the doctor's office. They represent one of the best "physical examinations" on Earth and can be performed without ever stepping a foot into a doctor's office. If you don't want to purchase these tests, simply do the free tests listed first. Then, at the end of three weeks, retest yourself and measure your progress. If the symptoms are gone and all markers are now in a normal range, you can begin to experiment with "cheating" from the program. Cheating, which basically means straying from synchronizing with one of the elements or eating processed foods, is often a good reminder of why you started this in the first place. Often people need to stray multiple times before they're convinced that this is the way to live to keep Whole Body Health. For the first three weeks, *do not cheat.* If you cheat, you need to start the program over again from the beginning. If you want to activate the power of this formula, you must follow it to the letter.

Tests to gauge your progress. In three weeks retest all of these tests as it takes longer to change and measure your progress.

1. Write out the four main symptoms that bother you:
   1. pain
   2. fatigue
   3. memory
   4. brain fog

2. Take your blood pressure, while reclining, then stand up immediately and take it again.

80

B.P. reclining _____. Pulse _____
B.P. Standing _____. Pulse _____
(Blood pressure should be under 130/90 and should
rise slightly on standing)

3. Mineral Cuff test - fill up B.P. Cuff around your
calf. Stop when the calf begins to cramp and write
down how high the B.P. was when this occurs.
     B.P. Cuff tests. _____
(Calf shouldn't cramp until 220mm of mercury, less
than this is a sign of a tissue mineral deficiency)

4. pH of the saliva taken for five mornings and
averaged _____
(Normal pH of the saliva is 7.2, anything below 7 is a
sign of acidity)

5. Breathe in and out several times and then hold
your breath as long as you're able. How long were
you able to hold it? _____ 25sec .
(Breath holding time should be at least 1 minute.
Anything less than 30 seconds is a sign of severe
acidosis of the body)

6. Put 2% Potassium Iodine on the skin in a two-inch
patch. Watch to see how long it takes to disappear. It
should take 24 hours, anything less is a sign of
deficiency. How long did yours take? _____

7. Waist Hip Ratio (WHR). Measure the
circumference of your belly at the widest point and
then your hips at the widest point. Then divide your
Waist inches by your Hip inches.
Waste circumference _____ /
Hip circumference _____ = ____|_____
(The World Health Organization defines anything

81

above a .90 for males and .85 for females as obesity)

8. Weigh yourself _____

9. Measure your waking body temperature every morning upon rising for five days. Then average the temperature and write it down. _____
(Anything below 98 is a sign of a slow metabolism and possible endocrine dysfunction)

10. Get blood work for the following:
Lipids - HDL, LDL, Total Cholesterol, triglycerides
Vitamin D   (Ideal - 50-70 ng/ml)
B-12   (Ideal - > 450 ng/L)
C-Reactive Protein.   (Ideal - < 1 mg/L)
HBG-A1C   (Ideal < 1 mg/L)
Glucose   (Ideal - 70-80 mg/dl)
TSH   (Ideal - < 2)
T3   (Ideal 3.7 - 4.2 pg/ml)
T4   (Ideal 6.0 - 12 mg/dl)
TPO   (Ideal < 4 IU/ML)

9 - HEALING THE MIND

REMOVE: Negative thinking and the curses in your life.
ADD IN: A power statement of healing and the reasons why you're going to always make the right choice and follow through.

"It has been verified through scientific exploration that more than 80 percent of all diseases are due to stress and strain that originate in the mind and reflect on the body".
—American Medical Association

Before we can talk about the body, we need to talk about the mind. In all my years of practicing, I have found that there are two types of patients that never get well. The first type are those that are being cursed, either by their own thoughts or by someone in power over them. Because of these curses they don't believe that they can get well and therefore either don't try or mentally sabotage any treatment received. The second type are those that don't have either a really good reason to get well or purpose for health. As soon as a healing protocol gets hard they quit because they never really had a good reason for doing it in the first place.

On the flip side, I have found that people with a strong purpose for healing follow the program and get healthy. A healthy mental state is necessary when it comes to healing and is called the power of the mind. Medical science calls this the placebo effect and it's documented to be as powerful as any medication. Spiritual leaders call it faith and the Bible states "For as a man thinketh in his heart, so is he." Success teachers call it the law of attraction, and even quantum physics confirm the incredible power of the brain.

It doesn't matter what you call it, it all means the same—What we think determines what our health will become, and the story that we tell ourselves will *probably* come true. Pir Viliyat Kahn said it best: "How we long to become that which we hardly believe we are."

The point of this chapter is to help you get your mind right so you have a chance at healing. By using the simple techniques described in this chapter, you can overcome the mental barriers between you and wellness.

While this may sound silly, this is the necessary first step in healing and cannot be skipped. There are three simple methods proven to put you in the right state to activate healing.

#1 - Reject the negative thoughts that come into your mind and the curses of those around.

` #2 - Find your purpose to heal, so that you never give up. When you feel like quitting (which you will at times) review your purpose, then continue with the proper action no matter how difficult it seems. Always take one more step in the right direction.

#3 - Bless yourself daily. Write out a power statement/prayer over your life. Repeat this at least twice daily when you wake up and before you go to bed. Never skip a day.

#1. REJECT THE CURSES

The story we've created in our mind is molded by the people we surround ourselves with, our experiences, and our daily thoughts. We especially believe the story we're told by those who have influence over us. Unfortunately, often the image created is a curse destroying our hope of healing. It can be a curse from our own thoughts, a curse from a loved one, or even a physician. For example, have you ever looked in the mirror and said "I feel terrible and I'm never going to get better?" Guess what you're doing? You are cursing yourself and your cells will hear you.

I get infuriated with doctors when they curse people with negative diagnosis such as, "You have fibromyalgia, and you will have it the rest of your life." Or the ultimate curse, "You have a terminal illness and six months to live." You must recognize this is a curse and refute both it and the doctor who says it.

The similarity between hospitals and churches is uncanny. Both are grand structures that house people in white robes who are in a position of authority. If you attend a hospital, after a long wait in the outer sanctum you gain access to the inner sanctuary where the doctor in his white robes divines your fate, often making you feel inferior since you don't understand the big words from his lexicon. Medicine, just like the ancient church, puts most diagnoses in Latin (a dead language) purposely so you don't understand what they mean.

"You have six months and then you will die unless you take these drugs," they might say. *Reject these curses*! Avoid any doctor who gives you a diagnosis (a curse) and prescribes a dangerous medication for life. This is witchcraft. In fact the word pharmacy comes from the Latin word *pharmacia* which literally means witchcraft.

Others curse us through their judgements of us or how we choose to live our lives. We might have had insensitive or abusive parents, or a spouse that berates us. Studies have shown that the combination of emotional stressors and low social support relate to a 9-fold increase in cancer.[61] This is documented to be one of the most powerful indicators in all disease, especially cancer. Emotional stressors must be resolved. Deepak Chopra in his book *Quantum Healing* states that the one thing that the remission of terminal cancer patients all have in common is a transformation of their mental attitude. It's the same for all diseases.

The first step in rejecting these curses is to become aware of your own thoughts and the words of those who surround you. Are they building you up or tearing you down? Are you smiling internally or screaming? Is your internal voice telling you about a future of happiness, love, and health, or is it constantly bombarding you with negativity?

Don't be a prisoner of the negativity surrounding you. Reject the negative thoughts. You can make that decision right now. Quit believing the lie and remove anyone from your life that is reinforcing this lie. If this an unemotionally supportive spouse, friend, parent or doctor, have a heartfelt conversation with them to seek their support. If you don't receive that support, then leave or fire them. Or stay and be sick, it's your life. There is no easy way of saying this and I know it's hard, but this is the core of many of our illnesses. By first becoming aware of negative thoughts, then actively replacing those thoughts with a new set, you can reprogram your mind. The next two steps will teach you how to accomplish this.

#2. FINDING YOUR PURPOSE

When a patient decides to come see me, I engage them in a deep and revealing conversation. I let them tell me their entire story. I listen and encourage them. Usually they are kind enough to open up and tell me their complete history. Once they're done sharing, I ask them, "Why do you need to resolve your health issue?"

I ask them this so I can find out their true motivation for healing. Often, I have to gently prod it out of them but usually they'll reveal their purpose for regaining health. If I hear answers such as, "I'm a single mother of two little children and I *need* to stay healthy so that I can help them grow up and make the most of their life," or "I'm going to Europe in six months and right now I don't have the ability or stamina to walk. I *need* to and will do *anything* to be able to walk through the streets with my spouse and enjoy this trip that we've dreamed about for many years." When I hear this, I say to myself, "Perfect! They are truly motivated to get better because they have a purpose."

If someone answers, "I don't know, my wife made the appointment. She's sick of hearing me complain about my pain." I cringe, because there is no real desire or intent to heal. Before you can take this WBH path, you must find your reason for wanting to take it. If you're just stumbling through the woods bouncing from path to path with no direction and no destination or reason for health, you will likely never find it. No matter what book you read, which doctor you visit, what health food store you shop at, you will never find it until you find your reason for it. This chapter on mind precedes all the other elements because the mind is the reservoir from which all health springs.

Many people genuinely want to get better and believe that they will. The problem arises because they are rather blasé about their success. As soon as healing gets hard, they quit and let the negative thinking slip back in. When questioned they kind of shake it off as it's not a big deal or find an excuse. Belief without willingness to do the work is useless. A desire for health with the inability to do what needs to be done to get healthy is worthless. Following the steps of this book is not easy; it's going to be hard and you will want to quit. This is the moment of truth for most people and is the difference between successful people and failures, between those who get well or remain ill. What is going to motivate you to make the right choice, every time?

When someone offers you a beer or a piece of pie, or you don't feel like getting up in the morning to do your routine, what is going to motivate you to push through toward Whole Body Health?

Tony Robbins, the famous motivational speaker, frequently talks about this but he calls it the *pain/pleasure* question. He says whatever is stronger in our minds, pain or pleasure, at any given minute about any choice that needs to be made, we will usually do. For example, if the pleasure of eating that donut outweighs the perceived pain that will come from it later, you'll eat the donut every time. On the other hand, if you associate eating the donut with massive pain, like the idea you're abandoning your children, gaining weight and destroying your life, you'll pass on the donut every time. Most of us will do more to avoid pain than we will to seek pleasure, so make sure the negatives associated with failure are strong enough to motivate your every action. By organizing your mind and thoughts, you can create a very clear image and associate your greater purpose with making the right health choices.

To achieve this organization of mind, Robbins conducts an effective exercise. He has people write down all positive future events that will make them feel absolutely happy and fantastic, a life fulfilled with purpose, that brings total and unabashed joy *if they follow through*. In a parallel column he has people write down all the terrible effects of failures and the absolute horrible feelings of a life destroyed *if they quit*. He has them use extreme emotions as a motivator to accomplish their purpose. Only with a powerful reason can you do the work to heal.

A story that impacted me deeply that further proves this point of a positive mental state and purpose is Victor Frankl's book *Man's Search for Meaning*. Frankl was a psychologist and a prisoner in the Auschwitz concentration camp during World War II. In his observations, he found that only about 1 in every 20 fellow prisoners survived, and he connected the ability to survive with a sense of purpose toward the future. From this observation, he sought to answer the question, "How was everyday life in the concentration camp reflected in the mind of the average prisoner?" This can easily be translated into, "how does life with illness affect a person's mental outlook?"

He found he could motivate his fellow prisoners to change their mental state, thus improving their chances of survival, by teaching the men how to imagine a life where they maintained a sense of purpose. The purpose could be something as simple as needing to do what only they could do, such as be a parent to a child. He admitted he survived from the desire/need to share his observations and psychology with the world. He found, when people focused on purpose rather than despair, it influenced their daily decisions. This in turn, changed their mental outlook and extended their lifespan.

Lastly, he described what he believed was the true purpose of life and why we're here in the first place—to find love. He poetically describes it like this, "A thought transfixed me: for the first time in my life I saw the truth as it is set into song by so many poets, proclaimed as the final wisdom by so many thinkers. The truth— that love is the ultimate and the highest goal to which man can aspire. Then I grasped the meaning of the greatest secret that human poetry and human thought and belief have to impart: *The salvation of man is through love and in love.* I understood how a man who has nothing left in this world still may know bliss, be it only for a brief moment, in the contemplation of his beloved."

This is the most important part of the book. Work to find your sufficient purpose to get well and learn to love yourself. Why *must* you pass on that donut *every* time. What is your purpose for healing and why *must* you accomplish it? Write it out right now.

Why *must* you get your health back and what is your purpose for doing so? List all the good things in your life that will happen if you gain back your health? Do it now!

What is going to happen if you don't get healthy? List all the bad and depressing things that will occur in your life if you give up and quit.

This exercise will help you reprogram your subconscious. The more extreme and vivid you are in your description, the more likely you will strive to avoid the negative condition and to obtain your highest goal. The person who clearly sees their new body, removes all negativity and doubt and then fuels that belief with unending action is the person who will achieve it, without exception. Put this list up somewhere you can see it every day!

#3. NOW, BLESS YOURSELF DAILY

"Believe that all the resources you need are in your mind. That is a formula that really works!"
—Norman Vincent Peale

Researchers have long known the power of placebo in medical outcomes. A 2001 meta-analysis concluded that the placebo effect can exceed the effect of active treatment by 20%.[62]

When approving a medication, the FDA only wants to see that it's slightly more effective than placebo to approve the medication. To activate the therapies suggested in the following pages you must believe that they will heal you. If you go into this saying, "I guess I'll give it a try for a little while," or "I bet this won't work but I need to do something," you have already sabotaged the program. You must believe with all your heart that you will be healed and give thanks ahead of time for that healing. A sick mind with self-defeating thoughts attracts breakdowns and sickness. A sick body attracts bacteria, virus, parasites, and disease of all kinds.

Fortunately, the opposite is true. A healthy body maintains immunity and a well-balanced environment for healthy function. A healthy mind with positive thoughts feeds the body with waves of wellness. Every cell in your body is listening to your thoughts. What are you telling them?

Studies have shown that the best way to activate this power of placebo is through repetition of positive words. The Bible says "pray with a grateful heart." So the obvious first step in healing is to come up with your power statement/prayer of being thankful for your victory over your condition. Are you going to get well or not? Decide right now. What is your positive placebo prayer for healing?

The ancients understood the concept of blessings. A Bible story that conveys the power of blessing is the story of Esau and Jacob. Esau was the elder brother and according to custom the rightful heir of his father's land, flocks, and most importantly his blessing of a good life. Their father was old and blind, and the day of the blessing was fast approaching. Being the youngest, Jacob was out of luck. However, his clever mother favored him, and schemed up a brilliant plan to help Jacob steal Esau's blessing. On the day that Esau was supposed to receive his blessing, Jacob's mother dressed him in Esau's furs. His mother made a meal and Jacob brought it to his dying and blind father. Upon entering his father's tent, his father asked, "Esau, is that you?" "Yes," replied Jacob. His father wasn't sure, for it seemed to him that Esau's voice was different. His father asked him to come closer and get down on one knee. His father kissed him, and sniffed to smell him. Esau's furs that covered Jacob did the trick. The old man smelled who he thought was Esau. Convinced that it truly was Esau, he blessed him: I bless you, "May God help you," he said. "May you have good crops and plenty of grain and wine. May you rule over other nations, and the rest of your family."

A few minutes later Esau came in looking for the blessing. Isaac said, "Your brother tricked me, I have given him your blessing." Esau pleaded, give me a blessing too dad, but Isaac said, "I am sorry Esau, I have no more blessings. Jacob has stolen them." Esau, being the elder and more powerful man, did not give up his lands or cattle, but it was the blessing that he lost out on, and he would have traded it for everything else. This is how much the ancients valued words. The truth is that words matter greatly. The words that we say to ourselves or others say to us very much determine our reality. It's imperative to healing that we rid our mind of negative words both from our own thoughts and the words that others speak to us.

When the negative thoughts creep back in, repeat your power statement over and over again. **Positive thoughts and negative thoughts cannot co-exist, so by repeating positive thoughts of healing, you will push out the negative.** This is such an important concept. We all have negativity floating around our brains—thoughts of disease and pain. The only way to overcome these thoughts is to reprogram your brain with positive statements. Say it over and over again with great feeling. Your brain might tell you in the beginning, "this is stupid" and "who are you kidding?" but keep saying it. Do this as many times per day as you can—say it when you first wake up and again when you go to bed. Constantly remind yourself that you are healed, activate the power of the mind, and then follow the steps laid out in this book and soon, I promise, you will be healed.

You can activate the power of placebo/faith/secret and learn to achieve self-love by blessing yourself daily. Write out your power statement right now. I have written out an example. Please copy it, modify it, or create your own, but make the last line the same as mine, "I am perfect, and I love myself completely."

Repeating this power statement, especially the last line, will move you towards WBH. As you learn to love yourself you will overcome your feelings of not being loved or accepted by others. With an improved self-image, you will be able to, maybe for the first time in your life, let go of the pain.

Every day you need to read this statement when you first wake up and right before you go to bed:

"I am so thankful that every cell of my body is fully and completely healthy and functioning perfectly, and that therapies I'm doing will heal me. I here and now commit to letting go of past curses, thoughts, and diagnoses and allow those to flow out of my body as they are not me. I will be aware of my thoughts and refuse any thoughts that do not match my new state of being of health. I choose to replace these dark thoughts with feelings of gratitude and a strong sense of purpose, which is,

_____

_____
_____
_____
_____
_____

_____." (Fill in your major life purpose.) I am sending light and love to every cell of my body. (Now visualize your entire body filling with light and love and don't stop until you feel like your entire body is full of light). I will repeat this process twice daily until I have achieved the self-confidence to know that *I am perfect, I am healed, and I love myself completely.*"

OK, you got your mind right, now you're ready! Let's activate.

10 - THE CARBOHYDRATE RESET

ELEMENT EARTH:

REMOVE: All carbohydrates and processed food
ADD IN: Organic healthy fat, vegetables, and meat

"When a food manufacturer sells you a denatured (processed) product, he is shortening your life for his profit. It is your responsibility to become sufficiently alert to prevent this from happening, and your patients depend on you for reliable information". —Dr. Royal Lee, January 1943

Now that your mind is right, let's activate the formula and move on to the *Earth* element. The most obvious first part of this element is dialing in which foods we're selecting from the Earth. The majority of us are consuming vast quantities of sugar, processed carbs, GMO grains, food colorings and a host of man-made chemicals. Unbelievably, 70% of the foods Americans consume are processed, high-carbohydrate foods. The average American is getting over 14 pounds of food additives[63] and over 150 pounds of sugar per year. This must change if we want to regain health. While most of us realize that a diet change is necessary, few comprehend how important it is when it comes to eliminating disease. Fewer still understand how our diet is affecting our energy production and how almost 100% of Americans are overeating carbohydrates and sugar.

In this chapter you'll learn how our bodies begin having multiple system breakdowns when we hit or exceed our daily carbohydrate max consumption. Our bodies morbidly convert from burning fat efficiently to burning sugar inefficiently. You're also going to learn the history of refined sugar, why I call it an *anti*-nutrient/ mineral, and how it's affecting us. Finally, you're going to learn to find your own carbohydrate max intake that your body can tolerate, allowing you to dial in the perfect diet. This chapter is a real eye-opener, full of "a-ha" moments, so hang on and enjoy the ride. Because there is some higher-end medical science, I'm going to make a few jokes and silly analogies to try to lighten it up and help get the point across.

SUGAR & CARBOHYDRATES

Processed carbohydrate foods are poison, plain and simple. These are the first thing that need to be removed as part of Whole Body Health. Webster's defines a poison as a "substance that through its chemical action usually kills, injures, or impairs an organism."[64] Controlled tests done on all processed foods prove that they injure, impair and kill us, therefore making it the very definition of poison. An old joke is, "how do you stop a man from drowning" The answer? You take your foot off of his head. If you are eating excessive sugar and refined carbohydrates, you are drowning in poor health, and the only solution to start rebuilding your health is to quit it completely.

Weston A. Price, in his travels, repeatedly found and documented that the consumption of sugar and refined carbohydrates was the primary attributing factor to the destruction of overall health in all human cultures. When it showed up in a territory, it invariably led to tooth decay and addiction. He carefully documented the subsequent decrease in health of societies. He found that with each generation that consumed refined carbs and sugar, they progressively became weaker and sicker. The decreased wellness was clear to detect, and the suffering it caused was apparent. Besides cavities, he

96

found soaring rates of tuberculosis, arthritis, depression and suicide. Dr. Price referred to these as "the disease of modern commerce." Later diseases like cancer, obesity and heart disease have been added to these diseases of modern commerce.

The goal of the next 21 days is to break the carbohydrate and sugar addiction, turn your body from a sugar burning, nutrient deficient, inflammation body to a fat burning, nutrient dense, low inflammation body.

Many people ask, as soon I tell them to quit carbs and processed foods, "*If they are so bad, why do I crave them so much?*" My answer is, "They're tasty, that's why!" Our evolutionary minds cannot get enough of this sweet stuff. This is what drove humans to the ends of the Earth in search of sugar. The reason humans are so bonkers for sugar and carbs is because they're so darn delicious. They are delicious because we're evolutionarily programmed to love and be full on addicted to sweetness.

This sweetness represents high-octane-fuel which the body can burn immediately, temporarily boosting energy. Our brain instinctively knows the value of quick energy so it turns on the pleasure part to keep us going back for more. To the Paleolithic man, sugar and carbs meant survival. It was the energy we needed to fight saber-toothed tigers. Additionally, sugary and carb foods in nature are almost never poisonous, while bitter foods often contain poison. It was bred into us as a survival instinct that sweet foods were safe to eat.

This sugar addiction drove us to harness sugar and inspired our brains to figure as many ways as we can to get more of it. Early on our ancestors would gather sweet foods in nature such as berries, honey, and fruit. It then led us to tapping maple trees for syrup, keeping bees in hives to harvest their honey, and horticulture of orchards of delicious sweet fruits like figs and apples.

And of course we fermented and distilled all of it into alcohol.

So when early humans came across sugar, such as a fruit tree or a beehive, they gorged on it until they couldn't eat another bite. Overconsumption was impossible as it would induce sickness and vomiting. In fact, the Bible admonishes us for overeating honey in Proverbs 25, "If you find honey, eat just enough—too much of it, and you will vomit."

The first historical step of sugar refinement was molasses, as it was much easier to ship it in this form. Molasses, while moderately high in glucose, is not a refined product and therefore it preserves nutritional value. If you eat too much molasses, like honey, you'll vomit. Due to this, it is difficult, if not impossible, to get diabetes from its consumption. Molasses (especially blackstrap) is rich in peptides, calcium, magnesium and iron, promoting healthy blood, hair, and bowel function. In addition to molasses, honey, jams, and most of the food sweetness was found congruently with nutrient density. As cultures' need to fight saber-toothed tigers disappeared, our insatiable yearning for sugar only increased.

THE PROBLEM

The real trouble came when sugar and flour were refined to its white crystal form now found on most supermarket shelves. Once the fiber and nutrients are gone, so too is our evolutionary brake that tells us we're full. "No vomiting you say? I think I'll eat the entire carton of ice cream, thank you very much."

Empty, refined carbohydrate consumption is by far the greatest threat to American health today. In fact, most Americans are getting a majority of their calories from sugar. The mass consumption of this white food is creating a nation full of sick people.

Refined carbohydrates are, as the name states, refined. The end result is a white food product. Sugars are anything that ends with "ose," such as fructose, lactose, dextrose, sucrose and are usually white. These sugars are known in the nutritional world as the twin white devils—white sugar and white flour. Make no mistake, when you eat white bread, you are eating sugar. The second it enters your mouth it's converted into sugar. I know this is devastating news for any Subway dieters.

Refinement removes all nutrition changing them to *anti-nutrient/anti-minerals* (ANTI). The term ANTI is for food that actually steals minerals from your body. These ANTI-foods quickly use up nutrient reserves to digest them. This net negative-nutrient eating depletes health reserves by borrowing nutrients and minerals from muscles, organs, bones, and teeth.

ANTI sugars shut off the "satiety hormone" called Leptin. Leptin is produced by the fat cells to signal to your brain and nervous system that you have enough fat reserves and should quit eating. Without leptin, you just keep on eating and eating and never feel full. Until we fill the nutritional gap caused by the ANTI-refined sugar, Leptin never tells us we're full. Since that day never comes for most us, we consume way too many calories, while at the same time starving for nutrition.

In 1950, Roger Williams published a paper in the *Lancet* called "The Concept of Genotrophic Disease."[65] He stated heart disease, cancer, arthritis, schizophrenia, and alcoholism could be considered genotrophic origins from under-nutrition (caused by sugar consumption) resulting in suboptimal metabolism and chronic illness. He was right, and it has gotten a lot worse in the last 65 years.

If you put a glass of Coke or Pepsi into 10 gallons of water, the pH will drop from 7.8 to 4.6 immediately. But, if the pH of our blood swings even 1 point either way, death is certain. Even if you drink 10 Cokes, the four to five liters of blood in our body must be maintained at 7.2.[66] How is this possible?

The way the blood pH never changes when consuming sugar is by sacrificing every other tissue. Calcium, magnesium, potassium and other alkaline minerals like chromium are sacrificed to buffer sugar's effects, and that's why a can of Coke doesn't kill us immediately. Thus the ANTI-nutrient/mineral aspect of sugar. These minerals are essential for cellular function, relaxation, brain chemistry, and bone health. Nobel Prize winner Linus Pauling stated that every disease can be connected to a mineral deficiency. The problem with sugar is that it is the great robber of minerals.

The Coke drinkers and sugar eaters of today will be the denture-wearing osteoperotics of tomorrow. I frequently see people in their 30s with the same bone density as 50-year-olds at my clinic. The problem is reaching the tipping point in our society.

Chronic sugar exposure makes all the cells and fluids of the body acidic as they give up their alkalizing minerals to buffer sugar. Robert Young in his book *The pH Miracle* discusses the importance of proper levels of pH at the cellular level. Out of whack, acidic pH levels make your body a breeding ground for parasites, bad bacteria, viruses, and candida. The acidic medium also contributes to cancer, heart disease, diabetes, osteoporosis, and heartburn.

Humans have crystalized sugar down to its most diabolically ANTI-refined form, high fructose. This process is akin to chewing coca leaves (molasses), turning it into cocaine (white sugar), then refining it into crack cocaine (corn syrup), and then refining it further into some sort of ludicrous super-spiked-crack cocaine (high fructose corn syrup). Seven billion crack addicted humans are attempting to quench an insatiable sweet tooth created by the very thing that created the addiction—refined sugar.

High fructose sugar has been shown in studies to create insulin resistance and fatty liver, damage intestinal bacteria, and cause metabolic syndrome.[67] It does this by creating an immune-mediated response[68] by helping endotoxins slip through the gut wall into the bloodstream, creating leaky gut. All this happens because fructose is poison and enormously inflammatory.

All that's left after the refinement process is insanely sweet poison devoid of any nutritional value. The manufacturers, in an attempt to market the products, then "enrich" it by injecting and spraying it with man-made vitamin compounds.

This enrichment process is akin to someone knocking you over and stealing $100 from your wallet then giving you back $100 in Monopoly money. Man-made vitamins do not work in the body as nutrients from organic food. This has been known for well over 100 years.

These isolated man-made vitamins don't work in the body, and in the end cause even more disruption to your health. Judith DeCava, in the article she wrote from Nutrition News, put it best:[69]

"Nature does not produce vitamins, minerals, trace minerals, or any other food components in concentrated or segregated forms, but merges and blends them— synchronizes them—for the body's needs. The idea that if a little is good, more is better leads to ingestion of mega-doses of 'high potency,' refined, separated

101

'nutrients,' dismantled, disassembled, or artificially manufactured chemical supplements. This will 'work' for a short time—pharmacologically stimulating or suppressing. Eventually, this method backfires and causes complications, imbalances. The body works to eliminate the excess and what it perceives as foreign, non-food. It attempts to combine the isolated chemical and other members of the complex, which normally appear in food, taking rather than giving. Such supplements do not contribute to health, they only disrupt it. Balance and function—not quantity—are the keys."

The sugar industry is fully aware of the addictive and disease-causing nature of these foods. The refinement of sugar creates one of the most highly addictive substances on Earth. This is the reason that it's included in almost every processed product today (ketchup, sauces, drinks, etc.). They want us addicted to their food so we keep on buying. The end cost is humanity's collective quality of life.

THE SCIENCE OF WHY CARBOHYDRATES ACTUALLY STEAL ENERGY

The second reason sugar and carbohydrates are so bad is that it's not the fuel that our bodies evolved to use. The Paleo diet has popularized this concept. Our bodies' cells are designed to burn fat for fuel. Each cell in our body has a factory inside it known as the mitochondria. Each mitochondria has an engine within it that converts fat to energy. This is called the Krebs Cycle. Putting fat through the Krebs cycle produces way more energy than sugar. Just as the engine in our car requires gasoline and oil, the engine of our cells requires fat and nutrients.

When your body runs on sugar it's an *extremely* inefficient anaerobic process. Glycolysis (burning sugar) yields four ATP (units of energy) but requires two ATP to be completed, therefore giving you two ATP per molecule of glucose. Fatty acid conversion (FAT) yield is 131 ATP per molecule of fatty acid. The activation of the fatty acid requires two ATP for a net energy of 129 ATP per molecule of 16 carbon fatty acid. Longer-chain fatty acids yield even more. Steric acid, an 18 carbon molecule yields 146 ATP and a 20 carbon fatty acid yields 163 ATP. Saturated fats like butter and coconut oil have the longest fatty acid chains. Put simply, we get many more ATP (energy) for every molecule of fatty acid (FAT) compared to a molecule of glucose (sugar). It's much more efficient which is why we evolved to burn fat for fuel.

Eating a molecule of butter is therefore over 80x more efficient at giving us energy than eating a molecule of sugar. (The naysayers to this example will argue that fat is bigger and heavier, but even with that consideration we're still getting over 3x as much energy for the weight.[70])

You can potentially run your car on a mixture of homemade alcohol and grease from your frying pan, but it won't run for long. Trying to run your body's engine off of anything other than fat is going to result in a breakdown as well.

THE CARBOHYDRATE HORMONES

Let's examine what happens when we eat sugar and carbohydrates. Try to stay with me for a minute and I'll make this complicated issue quite simple for you to understand.

The body spikes insulin production upon consumption of these substances. Insulin is a hormone produced by the pancreas that pushes sugar into the cells. Insulin triggers a cellular response that stops fat from being used while sugar is in the system. All cells in the body are sensitive to insulin, therefore if we consume too much sugar we can get stuck in the no fat-burning phase.

When we're eating sugar, and therefore running on it, our bodies are constantly producing insulin to get it out of the blood. The first place it puts the sugar is in the liver in a form called glycogen (liver sugar). When the liver's glycogen reservoir is full it starts pushing it into all the cells of the body. Once they're full, the body converts the excess sugar to triglycerides and fat.

Scientists have proven that sugar damages your DNA. Epidemiologist Lisa Givannelli of the Department of Pharmacology in Florence, Italy performed a study on 71 healthy adults (48 men and 23 women) and measured them for DNA damage. Her findings showed that the more processed sugar (glucose) a person consumes, the more oxidative DNA damage occurs in the blood cells. In contrast, a diet high in vegetables and low in sugar produces less or no DNA damage.

This is true of children, too. Often parents feel like they are doing a good thing by feeding their children juice boxes as a healthy snack, but these are full of sugar. Too much insulin depresses growth hormones and brain development in children.

Melanie Smith M.N.S., R.D. and Fima Lifshitz, M.D. of the Department of Pediatrics at Maimonides Medical Center, studied fruit juice consumption in children. They found that children 14-17 months old who had below-average growth patterns consumed excessive fruit juice.[71] Don't poison your kids. Sugar is poison, even fruit juice sugar.

When a body is constantly consuming carbs, the cells over time become insulin resistant. It's sort of like if there is a white noise going on all the time. Eventually

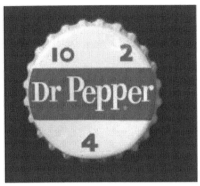

you quit hearing it, and you only realize it was there after it has been turned off. The same thing happens with the cells. When insulin is on all the time, the cells start to ignore it. This is called insulin resistance. The sugar has no place to go, so the pancreas desperately steps up the insulin to get it out of the blood.

Metaphorically, this process is similar to a parent asking their child to clean their room. At first they ask politely, and if the kid doesn't listen, they keep asking with greater urgency. Perhaps they keep calm for a while, but they come to a breaking point. If their unruly child continues to ignore them, they lose their temper and scream, "CLEAN YOUR ROOM NOW!" The kid finally pays attention, but by that time realizes that their room is so full of crap they don't know where to start.

The pancreas acts in the same manner. At first, it calmly does its job, sending a couple of warning signals telling the body's cells to accept this ready energy. But finally, as the cells can't accept more, it explodes with rage, screaming at your cells. The cells try to perk up and accept more sugar, but they're so full of soda and donuts, they just can't accept any more. Even a greedy kid can only eat so much pie. The parent screaming and overreacting is represented by the overproduction of insulin and the low blood sugar reaction that quickly follows.

Our irritability and fatigue created by this overreaction of our pancreas sends a signal to eat more sugar. Many people in our society feel these symptoms most acutely between meals around 10 am, 2 pm and 4 pm. Dr. Pepper knew this. They promoted this concept by putting on their label "best enjoyed at 10, 2 and 4." Dr. Pepper's marketing to these blood sugar drops is criminal genius. Dr. Pepper, along with the other soda cronies, are destroying humanity's health. Period.

I don't care if Dr. Pepper sues me for writing this. I hope they do. It'll be great marketing for the book, and I'll counter-sue them quicker than a one-legged man in an butt kickin' contest. They're terrified of the same class action lawsuits that the tobacco industry went through. Any lawyers reading this who want to make a billion dollars, these companies are an easy target. If you organize it, I'll be your first plaintiff.

If you completely cut out the sugar in your diet, glucagon, the opposite hormone to insulin, switches on. When glucagon is high we burn fat instead of sugar. Dr. Atkins had this figured out with his famous diet that massively limited carbohydrate consumption to increase glucagon. He knew high glucagon stabilized body weight and energy production. With high glucagon you will magically shed pounds, easily and automatically. The whole point of all this—quit eating sugar and carbohydrates.

A FEW MORE DEATH BLOWS BY SUGAR

DIABETES & ALZHEIMER'S

Diabetes is the next step of consuming too much sugar your body can't use. Eventually the sugar in your blood begins to rise. This is the crisis point and it gums up everything, including your vascular system, nervous system, and cellular function.

Adult-onset diabetes, also called Type II diabetes, is now being called childhood onset as so many children are becoming diabetic. Along with Type II diabetes, Alzheimer's is a direct result from this whole overconsumption of sugar. Some physicians and scientists are now calling Alzheimer's Type III diabetes. A cover story in *New Scientist* called, "Food for Thought: What You Eat May Be Killing Your Brain" covers how insulin helps keep the blood vessels that supply the brain healthy and encourages the brains neurons to absorb glucose. About 1/3 of Americans have diabetes or are close to having diabetes (pre-diabetic) resulting in Alzheimer's in old age.

Here's what best-selling author and neurologist Dr. David Perlmutter says in his groundbreaking book *Grain Brain:*

"[Alzheimer's] is a preventable disease. It surprises me at my core that no one's talking about the fact that so many of these devastating neurological problems are, in fact, modifiable based upon lifestyle choices... What we've crystallized it down to now, in essence, is that diets that are high in sugar and carbohydrates, and similarly diets that are low in fat, are devastating to the brain. When you have a diet that has carbohydrates in it, you are paving the way for Alzheimer's disease. I want to be super clear about that. Dietary carbohydrates lead to Alzheimer's disease. It's a pretty profound statement, but it's empowering nonetheless when we realize that we

107

control our diet. We control our choices, whether to favor fat or carbohydrates."

But nobody seems to be listening. By 2025, studies say that the number of people 65 and older with Alzheimer's disease will probably reach 7.1 million—40% more than 2015.[72]

This is my father's generation, and if I'm like most Americans, I'll just put him in an old person's prison, also called a nursing home. Every morning, he'll be fed more sugar in the form of orange juice and muffins and given endless medications. Medicare will pay the cost so his demise won't burden me. Out of sight, out of mind. Once a month I'll stop by with donuts and coffee for the underpaid staff and watch him drool for about an hour. I can justify this one, can't I? (Just joking, I love my dad and took him off all sugar!)

SUGAR AND THE TEETH

Weston A. Price documented that as sugar consumption goes up, pH drops and tooth decay begins immediately. Tooth enamel dissolves around a salivary pH of 5.5. Every time you eat sugar, the pH of your saliva drops to 4.5 and stays there for a 15 minutes. If you brush your teeth in this 15 minutes you literally can brush the enamel right off your teeth. Over time the weakened teeth soften, and cavities are formed. Brushing your teeth has never been the cure to tooth decay. Sugar is the whole story of decay.

SUGAR AND THE IMMUNE SYSTEM

Refined sugar lowers immune system response. I've used a live blood cell microscope and witnessed white blood cells go limp for 90 minutes after consumption of sugar, leaving your body wide open for disease. Since many of us are consuming sugar every 90 minutes, we are essentially living with permanently limp immune systems.

FREE RADICALS

Excess sugar in the blood also creates free radicals. Free radicals are like criminals in a society, too many of them overwhelm law and order. They destroy cells, arteries, and almost anything they encounter. By and large, free radicals are complete downers. Antioxidants and cholesterol protect us from them. Whole foods naturally contain antioxidants and nutrition to block free radical damage. If there aren't enough antioxidants around, cholesterol has to step up to repair the body. High cholesterol is a symptom rather than a core issue.

SUGAR AND THE GUT

Inevitably, not all sugar can be digested or pushed into the cells, so the excess has to be removed from the body. When the sugar reaches the colon, it destroys the good bacteria and promotes the bad bacteria called candida. We should have 7 to 8 pounds of good bacteria in our colons, resulting in around 100 trillion bacteria. In the digestion chapters, I cover this in much greater detail.

3 PHASES OF CARBOHYDRATE BREAKDOWN

The breakdown in the body due to excess carbohydrates follows a predictable pattern, and it's the same pattern of stress fatigue described in the first half of the book. First, it stresses our body, then it does damage, and finally it kills us. Each person consuming too many refined carbohydrates falls into one of the three categories. Traditionally it took until our 30s to reach phase I, mid 40s or 50s to reach phase II, and our

60s or 70s to reach phase III. More recently, we're seeing children in grade school in phase II and people in college reaching phase III.

CARBOHYDRATE BREAKDOWN SYNDROME

Take a moment to review the below phases and associated symptoms to determine what phase of the carbohydrate breakdown syndrome your body is in.

Phase I

1 Low energy (especially between meals at 10, 2, and 4—thanks Dr. Pepper).

2 Increased fat around the mid section of the body. This is the spare tire that is difficult or impossible to lose, caused by increased cortisol.

3 Blood sugar instabilities and the need to eat frequently. (Accompanied by irritability with skipped meals.)

4 Bloating and gas. Gas is never normal and a sign of carbohydrate fermentation occurring within the intestines.

5 Digestive issues of any kind.

6 Poor sleep (especially waking up between 1-4 in the morning).

7 Nervousness, Anxiety, Internal trembling, Depression.

8 Mental fog.

Phase II

1 More severe hormonal imbalances—infertility, menstrual irregularities, erectile dysfunction, etc.

2 Increased mental fog, anxiety, depression.

3 Increasingly poor energy (feeling tired and needing naps, with early afternoon being the most difficult).

4 Increased weight.

110

5 Increased insulin and glucose levels.

6 Increased blood pressure.

7 Increased digestive stress. (often people start having problems with heartburn, gall bladder pain and constipation).

8 Increased cholesterol.

9 Increased sleep issues—insomnia.

Phase III

√1 Obesity

2 Heart disease

3 Diabetes

?4 Alzheimer's

5 Cancer

√6 Mental Disease

√7 Endocrine Disease

√8 Chronic Fatigue

√9 Fibromyalgia

THE CARBOHYDRATE RESET

Yes, there is a solution and it's called the carbohydrate reset. It means that you quit *all* sugar for 21 days. Think about it—our ancestors often went long periods without sugar. In the summer and fall they would often feast on sugar. When it ran out, they would go into a natural state of ketosis in the winter and live off of hunting and root vegetables. This period of no sugar is a necessary reset for the body and should be performed yearly. A study published in *Cell Stem Cell*, at the University of Southern California, showed that long periods of this fasting shifts stem cells from a dormant state to a state of self-renewal and triggers regeneration of the system.[73]

By going completely off sugar for 21 days you literally reset how your body burns energy. When you don't have any sugar, your insulin levels drop and drain the built up sugar from your cells and liver. This allows glucagon (opposite hormone to insulin) to turn back on converting your body back into a fat burning machine.

The 21 day reset protocol breaks carb addiction because it completely eliminates all sugars. You need to be close to perfect during these 21 days and you cannot eat any carbs. If you slip and eat a donut on day 12, guess what? You have to start over. The first week of the reset will bring withdrawal symptoms for most of us and can be initially intense. This is called the "carb flu," and this response is no different from a crack addict going cold turkey. Remember, sugar addicts are essentially crack addicts, the ludicrous super-spiked-high-fructose-corn-syrup-crack-kind.

This reset is the only way to know for sure if sugar, carbs, and processed foods are a contributing factor to your symptoms. If the symptoms go away, presto, you figured out why you were sick—too many carbs and processed foods. This may be the most important "a-ha" moment of your life. Forever and always you will know what makes you feel bad.

For a long time, I've been influenced by a wonderful book and concept called the WHOLE30 by Dallas and Melissa Hartwig. They clearly build the case that carbohydrates are very bad. Other respected authors all said the same thing in their own unique way. They're all right: you must go on a carbohydrate fast to reset your health.

BOOKS EXPLAINING WHY WE NEED TO QUIT SUGAR AND CARBOHYDRATES

Sweet and Dangerous by John Yudkin M.D.
The Complete Scarsdale Medical Diet by Herman Tarnower
The Zone by Berry Sears
Sugar Busters by H.Leighton Steward, Morrison Bethea M.D., Sam Andrews, M.D., Luis Balart, M.D.
Atkins diet by Dr. Atkins
Eat fat, lose weight by Louise Gittleman M.S.
Eat fat, lose fat by Dr. Heyman
Eat fat and grow slim by Dr. Mackarness
Your fat can make you thin by Calvin Ezrin M.D.
Optimal Nutrition by Naj Kwasniewski
Eat Fat, Get thin by Barry Groves
Ducan Diet by Pierre Dukan
Paleo Solution by Rob Wolf

You will not get healthy unless you complete this step. This is the cornerstone of all future health decisions. Sound difficult? Sugar is arguably the most easily addicting substance on earth, so it will be hard to break its hold. You'll miss your favorite addictive industrialized junk food, but push through it. Cancer is difficult—you can do this!

Appendix A has a list of all foods allowed during the reset. You can prepare them however you like. My favorite is to simply cut up lots of vegetables and then bake them in the oven with lots of fat (coconut oil, butter, lard, olive oil, etc). If it's not on this list, don't eat it. For 21 days, you will eat like humans did for 99.9% of our evolutionary existence. Which basically means you can eat vegetables, fat and protein (if you choose)...and that's it!

AN ESSENTIAL EXERCISE—WRITE DOWN ALL OF YOUR SYMPTOMS

Write down all the symptoms your are experiencing before beginning this reset. Here are the most common symptoms that go away during the carbohydrate reset.

Symptoms:
✓ Bloating and gas
Indigestion
✓ Irritability and anger
✓ Low energy
✓ Brain fog
✓ Insomnia
High blood pressure
✓ Excess weight
✓✓ Body aches and pains

At the end of 21 days, look at the list and see which symptoms/complaints are gone. When you start eating carbohydrates again, try to determine how much you can tolerate before symptoms return. (i.e. weight gain, bloating, pain). Each of us has a carb tolerance number, sort of like the sleep number, and it is necessary that you figure out that number. Once symptoms return, lower your carbohydrate consumption below this amount.

A wonderful book called, *Life without Bread* by Christian Allen, Ph.D. and Wolfgang Lutz, M.D. studied the level of carbohydrates that most people can tolerate and found that the average max is 72 grams. There are lots of websites and apps for the phone that can help you manage this number. Get one and stick with it.

When deciding to bring carbohydrates back to your diet, know this: There are *no* essential carbohydrates needed for the body to function. 72 (average) grams is the max, the minimum is *none*. If you're not sure, don't eat it! Less is better. This number can add up quickly, since there are 72 grams in *one* bagel or *one* cup of dry cereal. Since there are some carbohydrates in other food too, it means that you cannot afford to eat *any* refined carbohydrates.

THE THREE-WEEK FIX

Cut out all carbohydrates and processed foods for three weeks to reset, then restrict all carbohydrates to a max 72 grams per day while trying to find your own tolerance level. Eat as much of other foods as you want.

QUESTIONS ABOUT THE 21 DAY CARBOHYDRATE RESET

Q. What if I get a week into this and go to my friend's party and eat cake? It's her birthday, and it's homemade and she uses the best organic ingredients.

A. No excuses. If you eat cake you will have failed the 21 day reset. Review your purpose for health, and then start over. You didn't complete the 21 days. There is no way to know which health issues are from sugar unless you go completely through the reset.

Q. What about coffee and alcohol?

A. No coffee or booze. Alcohol is in essence "insane sugar." It is partially fermented or distilled sugar that causes biochemical damage. Small amounts of alcohol are permitted once the 21 day reset is finished, if you like. My health didn't really begin to skyrocket until I finally accepted that I'm done with beer. It was the hardest and happiest day of my life.

115

Extremely acidic coffee borrows from your future health reserves by raising cortisol levels. Don't touch it for 21 days. (I love coffee and I know this is hard.) At the end of 21 days you can begin to drink *nuclear fusion coffee*. I came up with this coffee, which is based on the idea of bulletproof coffee, only much better. See appendix C for the recipe that you can begin to drink on day 22.

Are you going to have symptoms from the withdrawal? Probably, because you're addicted. It's a good thing to take a break. You may find when you're done with the 21 days you won't want it anymore. Wouldn't that be something!

Q. Can I eat fruit sugar? I mean, it's good for you.

A. No, don't eat it. None, not even the blueberries. Fruit is sugar. Yes, there are vitamins and enzymes in there. But it can wait for three weeks to reap the benefits of the 21 day reset. After the 21 days, low glycemic fruit like berries can be consumed. Sorry, I like bananas too, but not for the carb reset.

Q. This is hard. Are you sure this is a good idea?

A. I know it's hard, but so is being sick and living with health issues. If you're unwilling to go through the reset, you are not willing to heal yourself. If you can't find a good enough reason to rejuvenate the quality of your life, then *sayonara* my friend! Say hello to your doctor for me.

Q. Can I smoke?

A. Yes you can. Know that sugar issues are often the basis of other addictions. Once you reset, cigarettes might not be desirable anymore. This is the day you can quit. I have found many people can switch to an Indian tobacco known as Lobelia Inflata. Indian tobacco had none of the side effects of tobacco and actually helps clear the lungs. If you're smoking try smoking this first. You're going to need a pipe to smoke this so order that along with the herb. You can order this on Amazon.com.

Q. Can I use artificial sweeteners?

A. Hell no! Punch yourself in the face for asking that! (Kidding! Don't really punch yourself.) These are an even bigger problem than sugar. Sucralose, Sweet'N Low, and Aspartame are all much sweeter than sugar and are powerful neurological toxins. I even want you to avoid the so-called "healthy" fake sugars like Xylitol and Stevia. We're trying to break the sweetness addiction, so for a while it all has to go.

Q. Should I count calories?

A. Absolutely not, eat as much as you want. At this point in the program eat until you are full and completely satisfied. When you get hungry, eat again. The calorie in, calorie out formula is not even a little bit important during this phase. This phase is all about converting your body to burning fat for fuel and emptying your sugar reserves. As soon as your body switches to burning your own fat, you won't be hungry anymore.

Q. Don't I need carbohydrates for brain function?

A. Your brain does need between 150-200 grams of sugar daily, but it can be manufactured from amino acids and parts of fat through a process known as gluconeogenesis. So yes, you do need carbohydrates. But no, you don't need to eat them.

Q. What if I'm a vegetarian, can I still do this?

A. The word protein comes from the greek word meaning "of first importance:" There are eight essential amino acids: valine, lysine, threonine, leucine, isoleucine, tryptophan, phenylalanine, methionine. They are needed for your enzyme systems, muscles, cellular and metabolic functions. They must be in your diet because your body cannot produce them. You can be a vegetarian during the 21 day reset if you choose, but work to get plant proteins, and eat at least one egg per day.

Q. Can I overeat meat?

A. The human body was designed to be able to eat solely meat for long periods of time. Before refrigeration and canning most ancient people would spend the entire winter consuming only meat. In *My Life as an Indian* by J.W. Schultz says: "The Kutenais (Indians) brought with them large quantities of arrowroot and dried camas, the latter a yellow, sweet, sticky, roasted bulb which tasted too good to one who had not seen a vegetable of any kind for months." Healthy pastured meat, when digested properly, does not create acidity or mucus build-up in the body. The acid in meat is easily buffered and does not contribute to acidity in the body. Only sugar and nutritional deficiencies create acidity. Don't be confused, meat is ok. While you should try to fill most of your plate with 80% healthy vegetables, there is no limit on meat.

Unlike the Atkins diet, you don't need a diet of straight protein. Most of the foods you eat should be vegetables and fat. Listen to your body and eat what feels right. Pay attention to the details when eating protein. If it's beef, is it grass-fed? If it's dairy, is it grass-fed? How do you feel after I eat it? The protein that you do eat should definitely be organic.

Q. Is my energy going to drop?

A. The more your body is addicted to sugar and using it for energy, the more your energy is going to drop until it begins to burn fat. This is the famous carb flu. Your energy will only drop until your body remembers how to burn fat for energy. By replacing the carbohydrates with fat, it will provide all the energy and satisfaction that you need.

Q. Why is the reset 21 days long?

A. It takes 21 days to create a habit or break one. The concept of 21 days, or three session of seven days is powerful and even biblical. Daniel 10:3 speaks of abstaining from 'delicacies' and 'wine' for 21 days. 21 days gives your body a sufficient duration to drain sugar stored in the cells. Throughout the 21 day reset you will feel layers of dysfunction and disease melt away.

Q: Am I going to be completely healed after 21 days?

A: Maybe, maybe not. 21 days is the bare minimum to see if carbohydrates are creating your illness.

Q: Can I go back to eating like I did at the end of 21 days?

A. If after 21 days your health is much better, and you're asking this question, then go ahead and be sick again. It's your body and your life, but I wouldn't recommend it.

Q: What if I get constipated on a low-carbohydrate diet?

A: Constipation is common when beginning a low carbohydrate diet. This is a sign of toxicity of the bowels. The chapter on digestion discusses the treatment of the digestive system. If you are constipated, eat less meat and more vegetables. If you're still constipated do a daily enema with warm water. It will usually normalize within a week or two as your body becomes accustomed to the new diet and the muscles of your bowels strengthen.

OK, so now your diet is correct. It's time to reestablish the earth element within our bodies...

11 - MINERALS AND VITAMINS

ELEMENT EARTH

REMOVE: Non-organic produce and continue to avoid sugar
ADD IN: Minerals and vitamins

REPLACEMENT OF MINERALS and VITAMINS

"All living cells are like an idling automobile engine"
—Dr. Royal Lee

Minerals and vitamins act as spark plugs for our cellular engines. The millions of functions throughout the body's cells cannot happen without adequate minerals and vitamins. Trying to run your body without them is like asking the Ford factory to make cars without parts. Cells compose our entire body. We are, in reality, just a fluid filled bag of cells. All these cells are individual idling engines working together to create functions such as a muscle contraction to pick up a glass of water. A deficiency of minerals is found in every case of chronic disease and stress. This concept was noted by Linus Pauling, one of the original scientists of the Vitamin C molecule and two-time Nobel Laureate, when he emphatically stated, "One could trace every sickness, every disease and every ailment to a mineral deficiency." When I first began to meet physicians who were getting real results, they would often tell me "it's all about minerals when it comes to healing." They're all so right, and you're about to learn why.

121

This chapter is all about replenishing our reserves. As you should be completely aware by now, stress and *anti* sugar deplete our reserves until our tank is empty. In this chapter, you're going to learn why practically everyone is starving for nutrition, how it creates disease, how to test your own mineral levels, and finally the exact methodology for refilling your gas tank. We cover some remarkable ground, so strap yourself in and let's figure out how to replenish Earth's nutrients within us and maybe save the Earth along way...

There are 90 elements naturally occurring on Earth, 22 are essential to life, and these make up about 4% of our total weight. This is broken down into macro and micro elements. We need at least 100 mg/day of macro minerals in our food like calcium, phosphorus, magnesium, sodium, potassium...and less trace minerals. Sadly, because of sugar over-consumption and dead empty soil, almost 100% of people I measure are deficient in minerals. The following is an explanation of how and why our soil lost all of its mineral content and how to fix it.

SOIL AND MINERALS IN AMERICA.

The first settlers to America's Great Plains could barely believe their eyes upon seeing land with virgin topsoil under native, deep-rooted grass. The settlers would say, "In America, the streets are paved with gold!" This was a direct reference to the richness and fertility of the soil—black gold, they would say. The wealth and fertility of the American landscape was the foundation for the development of a powerful and prosperous society.

Sadly, there has been a dramatic loss of mineral-dense topsoil in the last 150 years. This is due solely to the profit-driven mega mono-agricultural and conventional farming methods.

Globally, for the last 100 years, our farming methods have revolved around extraction, and these extraction methods have depleted a majority of the topsoil and with it the nutritional density of the food it produces. Those same Great Plains settlers who discovered the deep, virgin topsoil proceeded to till it with deep plowing over many years, leading disastrously to the Dust Bowl of the 1930s. Tearing up those native grasses to excess, which trapped moisture and hosted microorganisms, destroyed a vast wealth of soil.

According to estimates, globally, we have about 60 years of topsoil left until we will no longer be able to grow crops if we continue to use the same monoculture extraction methods that are being widely used.[74] Volkert Englesman, an activist with the International Federation of Organic Agriculture, states "We are losing 30 soccer fields of soil every minute, mostly due to intensive farming."[75] The last few inches continue disappearing at a current rate of one percent per year.[76]

Petroleum-based fertilizers are the only 'return' the land receives. Neither bacteria, nor minerals, nor decomposing life are brought back into the cycle and the soil is never allowed to rest. The integral cycle of new soil creation is completely disrupted, leaving the soil devoid of life and nutrition.

You probably hear people discuss peak oil with its environmental and economic devastation, but you hear almost no one talking about guaranteed human extinction once the topsoil is gone. Peak soil, not peak oil, should be humanity's number one global concern.

The situation is dire, as only a few inches remain in fewer and fewer areas, stretching thin the possibility of a healthy, well-fed world. Unless there is a mass awakening, we face mass starvation and disease in the very near future.

SOIL AND DISEASE

The old statement "you are what we eat" rings true when it comes to minerals in the body. In the Bible, God famously forms Adam out of the dust of the Earth and states: "From dust we came, and dust we shall become." This is exactly right. The health of a society can be directly connected to the health of the soil—all diseases can be tracked to a deficiency of one of the minerals from the soil. Soil health is a mirror of the health of people living on that soil. One handful of healthy live soil contains seven billion organisms, the same population as humans on earth. It is a perfect balance of decomposition and new life. The same nutrients, minerals, vitamins and bacteria that make up the entire body can be found in one handful of healthy soil. As goes the soil, so goes the human cells—as goes the human cell, so goes the mind—as the mind goes, so goes society —as goes society, so goes the next generation. The ever-present thread holding it all together is healthy soil and minerals.

With the loss of rich topsoil, humans are progressively becoming more deficient and with that deficiency we are stressed and diseased. In fact, you can track any disease in humans to a deficiency of minerals. Here are some examples: If you live inland and there is no iodine in your soil, your thyroid cannot convert hormones properly and you may become depressed or overweight. If there is no zinc, you may develop liver disease and skin issues because it's needed to heal. If there is no chromium, cobalt nor nickel in the soil, your blood sugar cannot properly regulate and you'll likely develop diabetes or gain weight. If there is no magnesium, you will get heart disease. No calcium— osteoporosis: no trace minerals—cancer. And so it goes.

124

This is not a new problem. We knew as far back as 1936 that we were depleting the soil of minerals with our farming techniques. Senate Document no. 264, recorded in 1936, states "The alarming fact is that foods—fruits and vegetables and grains—now being raised on millions of acres of land that no longer contains enough of certain needed minerals, are starving us—no matter how much of them we eat!"

Laboratory tests prove that the fruits, vegetables, grains, eggs, and even the milk and meats of today are not what they were a few generations ago (which explains why our forefathers thrived on a selection of foods that would starve us). Nobody can eat enough fruits and vegetables to supply their system with sufficient minerals. Look at the chart comparing the mineral content of organically grown food to modern commercial foods. Look at the differences of mineral content in the chart.

PERCENTAGE OF DRY WEIGHT		MILLEQUIVALENTS PER 100 GRAMS DRY WEIGHT				TRACE ELEMENTS PARTS PER MILLION DRY WEIGHT				
Tot. Ash Mineral	Phosphorus	Calcium	Magnesium	Potassium	Sodium	Boron	Manganese	Iron	Copper	Cobalt
SNAP BEANS										
Organic	10.45	0.36	40.5	60	99.7	8.6	73	60	227	69	0.26
Commercial	4.04	0.22	15.5	14.8	29.1	0.9	10	2	10	3	0
CABBAGE										
Organic	10.38	0.38	60	43.6	148.3	20.4	42	13	94	48	0.15
Commercial	6.12	0.18	17.5	13.6	33.7	0.8	7	2	20	0.4	0
LETTUCE										
Organic	24.48	0.43	71	49.3	176.5	12.2	37	169	516	60	0.19
Commercial	7.01	0.22	16	13.1	53.7	0	6	1	9	3	0
TOMATOES										
Organic	14.2	0.35	23	59.2	148.3	6.5	36	68	1938	53	0.63
Commercial	6.07	0.16	4.5	4.5	58.8	0	3	1	1	0	0
SPINACH										
Organic	28.56	0.52	96	203.9	237	69.5	88	117	1584	32	0.25
Commercial	12.38	0.27	47.5	46.9	84.6	0.8	12	1	49	0.3	0.02

Dr. Charles Northern is one of the fathers of mineral research. He discovered and showed the following: "In the absence of minerals, vitamins have no function. Lacking vitamins, the system can make use of minerals, but lacking minerals vitamins are useless." Additionally: "Bear in mind that minerals are vital to human metabolism and health—and that no plant or animal can appropriate by itself any mineral which is not present in the soil upon which it feeds." He went on to write: "Neither does the layman realize that there may be a pronounced difference in both foods and soils—to him one vegetable, one glass of milk, or one egg is about the same as another. Dirt is dirt, too, and he assumes that by adding a little fertilizer to it, a satisfactory vegetable or fruit can be grown."

Our foods vary enormously in value, and some of them aren't worth eating. For example, vegetation grown in one part of the country may assay 1,100 parts per billion of iodine, versus 20 that are grown elsewhere. Processed milk has run anywhere from 362 parts per million of iodine and 127 of iron, down to nothing.

When the mineral levels drop in the food, so does the taste. Can you remember, for those older people, the incredible flavor of homegrown strawberries, tomatoes and corn? Once the minerals are lost, it tastes more flat. As a result, we're adding sugar to increase the flavor which only serves to deplete even more minerals.

Think about this. We are starving, no matter how much we eat. This is partially why we overeat. We eat and eat, but our body never turns off the appetite because it knows it's starving from mineral deprivation.

Without sufficient minerals, our digestion can't activate enzymes, vitamins have little function in the body, and our cells are unable to produce and maintain their electrical charge, needed to respond to stress. Without sufficient charge the metabolism of the body slows.

It's not just our bodies that are starving, so are our brains. Dr. Royal Lee called calcium, potassium, and iodine the soothers of the mind. As we see the mineral content dropping in our food, we're seeing a direct correlation with an increase in mental problems. It pains me to watch school lunchrooms feeding kids juice and high-carb sugar lunches. Then, because these poor kids have no minerals, their mental function drops, so we drug them with powerful medications that further numb their already stressed nervous systems. What are we doing?

Gibran's words from his masterpiece *The Prophet* describes our relationship to soil: "To you the earth yields her fruit, and you shall not want if you but know how to fill your hands. It is in exchanging the gifts of the earth that you shall find abundance and be satisfied. Yet unless the exchange be in love and kindly justice, it will but lead some to greed and others to hunger."

SOLUTIONS AND SUPPLEMENTATION

The solutions are many. It starts with understanding, and quickly spreads into action and support. We purchase and support only produce from small organic farms that are living in harmony with the land and therefore are imbibed with nutritional density. We avoid processed foods and sugars, knowing that these foods leech the minerals out of our bodies and the Earth. Only by eating like this can we have a chance to maintain our long-term health, recover from stress, and save the world. The best supplements in the world are always food. As you may have noticed, I haven't mentioned vitamins much. Don't worry about vitamin supplementation because only whole food vitamins work. Seek to eat more nutritionally and mineral dense foods.

The following list of organic foods are the densest source of the following minerals and vitamins:

- Calcium—Organic dairy, dark greens, bone broth
- Chromium—Organic brewer's yeast, grains, clams
- Copper—Organic oysters, organ meats, nuts
- Iodine—Organic and wild seafood
- Iron—Organic red meat, fish, green vegetables
- Magnesium—Organic green vegetables, nuts
- Manganese—Organic nuts, fruit
- Phosphorus—Organic meat, fish, poultry, eggs
- Selenium—Organic seafood, nuts, meats
- Zinc—Organic meat, liver, eggs, seafood

After we begin to eat like this, we can begin to supplement minerals. A good multi-mineral supplement should have at least 70 minerals present and must be chelated. The word chelated or organic (the terms are exchangeable) means that the minerals have been taken out of the soil by a plant and in the process had a protein attached to the mineral. When using truly chelated minerals, the size of the minerals are microscopic. They are around .00001 microns, which gives them enormous surface space to be absorbed. These minerals become negatively charged, which allows them to be absorbed by the small intestine. It's these minerals that have the ability to conduct an electrical current that all cellular function requires. Again, they are the spark plugs of the cell.

The problem arises in that same greedy thinking that resulted in the loss of soil. This same thinking drives the manufacture of supplements, which are often completely unusable by the body. Almost all man-made minerals, supplements come from inorganic and non-chelated compounds, which render them mostly indigestible. The vast majority of mineral supplements are inorganic compounds and made from ground-up rocks and oyster shells.

So I just laugh when I see a brand of antacid like TUMS advertising that they are now adding calcium carbonate to their products. The function of TUMS is to lower acidity of the stomach, thus hampering mineral absorption in the first place (you'll learn about this in the next chapter). Then they add calcium carbonate which is just ground up rock. The only possible result of consuming this "supplement" is a kidney stone. In my practice, Whole Body Health, we routinely measure vitamin and mineral content by measuring cellular function. We do this by measuring the patient on a medical bio-impedance scale. This is how I measure the cellular charge that I described in the first half of the book. The three things this scale shows me are phase angle, capacitance, and intra- and extra-cellular water. The three tests measure the cellular charge, the level of cell breakdown, and the water composition of the cell. This is a wonderful way to quickly assess cellular terrain and patient health.

At any time, 60% of the water in the body should be inside the cells. If it's less, it indicates chronic dehydration and therefore lack of function of the cells. The Phase Angle measures the cell breakdown. Just like in soil, there should be a constant circle of breakdown and creation of cells; too much breakdown indicates a problem. The capacitance is the energy gradient from the intra- and extra-cellular membranes—basically the electric potential of the cells.

So when I see someone that has accelerated cell breakdown, low-energy gradient and dehydration of the cells, what I'm witnessing is the death of a human right in front of my eyes. These people always have acidic saliva accompanying the previous tests described, as both are signs of deep levels of mineral deficiency. To restore health, mineral supplementation must occur. So let's learn how to test and supplement ourselves.

TESTING

Testing which minerals are deficient in our body and replacing them is quite easy, if not quick. Each of us can easily and cheaply measure our saliva pH as an indicator of overall mineral health. Normal pH of the saliva should remain around a 7.2. It's most accurate to check your pH in the morning before you've eaten any food. I recommend that you measure your pH for several days to get an average. Use this method:

Whole Body Health pH Analysis

1.Measure your saliva first thing in the morning, before eating or drinking.

2.Record the pH on the chart below in each box, respectively, for the next seven days. Then average the seven days and write it down. The pH should be slightly alkaline.

pH saliva	Day 1	Day 2	Day 3	Day 4	Day 5	Day 6	Day 7
5.5							
5.8							
6.0							
6.2							
6.4							
6.6							
6.8							
7.0							
7.2							
7.4							
7.6							

AVERAGE PH _____

If your average salivary pH is acidic, then in addition to cutting out sugar you must supplement minerals. The fastest and most effective method I know for correcting the mineral imbalance and salivary pH is with Humic and Fulvic minerals.

HUMIC AND FULVIC MINERALS - BLACK GOLD

Fulvic acid occurs naturally as a derivative of decomposing humus (humic) plant matter. Humus is the decomposing part of healthy, bacteria-rich soil and serves many functions. Most importantly, plants use this to more easily chelate the minerals out of the soil. Without them, plants grow deficient in minerals. **These plants that are deficient in minerals become overly abundant in certain amino acids, which literally attract pests.** Farmers then make the same mistake that doctors make, instead of correcting the ninerals, they go after killing the pests with additional pesticides and insecticides. These in turn kill more of the humus, which results in a weaker next generation of the plants. This cycle of destroying the topsoil will continue until an awakening occurs.

Thankfully, there are deposits of Humic and Fulvic acids around the world that came from ancient, lush decomposing vegetation. Some of these deposits have remained near the surface so they didn't turn into coal or oil and are very high in Humic and Fulvic acid. While these deposits are quite rare, they are the most powerful way to reactivate healthy mineral function in the body. Think of it like treating your cells to diamonds and gold.

When I first became aware of Humic and Fulvic minerals and started experimenting with them, I believed that I had found the magical missing link in health. Why? Because they quickly reestablish cellular charge in the body. When ancient cultures found deposits of ancient Humic and Fulvic minerals they would refer to it as the "the gift" from Mother Earth.

These deposits are so powerful because they possess biologically-active electrolytes and contain within their structure over 60 minerals, supercharged antioxidants, nutrients and enzymes. The term, "biologically active" means that the Fulvic mineral electrolytes can reintroduce an electrical potential to human cells. The minerals can both act as an electron donor or an electron acceptor depending on the cell's requirements, making them able to recharge stressed cells.

As shown in the first half of the book, our cellular environment changes and the electrical charge drops when we're overly stressed. The cellular charge drops because of low minerals and then, just like plants, the cell walls rupture and attract pathogens (parasites, bacteria, virus, etc.) designed to clean them up. Various disease states are activated as the cellular charge continues to drop.

By using Fulvic minerals you can quickly charge your cells and provide minerals and vitamins needed to balance body chemistry. If the pH of your saliva averages less than 7.0, then you will be taking these minerals for the entire 21 day reset. At the end of 21 days, retest the pH of the saliva. If it's still acidic, then continue mineral supplementation.

OTHER INDIVIDUAL MINERALS THAT SHOULD BE CHECKED

There are a few minerals that we often need to supplement, including iodine, zinc and calcium/magnesium. These minerals play such an important role in the body that a deficiency will almost guarantee disease. Here's a quick explanation of each of these minerals and the simple home test you can use to see if you need to supplement them.

IODINE

Iodine is found mostly in the oceans and the soil that surrounds the oceans. It forms the basis of our metabolism and is the gas pedal of the cell. Once consumed, 80% of iodine is sequestered to the thyroid gland while the rest is mostly in the salivary glands, gastric mucosa, lactating mammary glands, and ovaries.

Years ago, doctors would immediately prescribe iodine for any symptoms of thyroid dysfunction and for any metabolic symptoms they didn't understand. Dr. Albert Szent Gyorge, Nobel Prize winning physician, said, "If you don't know where, what, and why prescribe ye then K and I(iodine)." Rockefeller Medicine quit using iodine when they developed synthetic thyroid hormone substitutes such as Synthroid and Levothyroxine. As you can imagine, the cheap and effective use of iodine was immediately abandoned for

133

the higher priced addictive substances. Iodine prescription was stripped from the medical curriculum and mostly forgotten.

Cultures that have a higher rate of iodine consumption have less obesity, less thyroid disease and less cancer—especially breast cancer. Unfortunately, most Americans have insufficient concentrations of iodine in their bodies.

The U.S. government realized this 100 years ago, and in the 1920's mandated the addition of iodine to salt because large quantities of people were getting goiters due to iodine deficiency. Despite this, iodine deficiency remains at a record high. The reasons are several. First, they add it to bleached, toxic white salt instead of real salt like sea salt or Himalayan salt. Second, the ubiquitous presence of toxic elements like chlorine and fluoride in our water have a lighter atomic weight and displace iodine, making supplementation essential.

The easiest, safest, and most effective way to measure iodine levels is to paint it on the skin of your forearm in about a two-inch square. This iodine should last 24 hours before fully disappearing. If it lasts less than 24 hours, your body is deficient and greedily "sucking" the iodine up like a thirsty person drinking water. Use the following graph to compare how long it takes to disappear.

HOW TO SUPPLEMENT IODINE

Many doctors propose taking mega doses of potassium iodine each day often in the range of 12-36 mg. This is about 24,000x the recommended dose. Don't fall into this trap. Remember, when we take high dose isolated minerals or vitamins, they have a drug-like effect and can create other dysfunctions in the body. I recommend taking a much smaller dose of between 150-600 micrograms per day. It frequently takes 6-12 months or more of supplementation to fill back up your iodine storage, so stick with it.

ZINC

Zinc is probably the most deficient single mineral in the world right now because modern farming techniques are quickly depleting it. Zinc is necessary for the immune and digestive systems, and for healthy liver function. It is especially important for pregnant women, as it helps prevent birth defects. Symptoms of zinc deficiency include:

White spots on the nails
Acne
Pale, dry skin

135

Dandruff
Slow wound healing
Low immune system
Poor digestion and leaky gut
Sex hormone disturbance

Zinc can be checked easily and accurately measured by using a zinc taste test. Standard Process Nutrient Labs has a good zinc taste test. Lack of a strong metallic taste is an indication of a zinc deficiency. If tasting the zinc produces a strong metallic taste then your zinc level is at a sufficient level. In testing my office performs, I've found that over 90% of people are deficient in zinc. Since zinc is necessary for enzyme activation and the healing of leaky gut, everyone should check their levels and supplement if needed.

CALCIUM/MAGNESIUM
America consumes among the most calcium of any nation on earth, yet we also suffer from the highest level of osteoporosis on earth. That's because many processed foods are fortified with calcium. The problem with this, as you may recall, is that these fortified foods utilize inorganic and mostly indigestible forms (remember TUMS) and they are not combining it with magnesium, which is necessary for proper utilization in the body. In the body, the calcium/magnesium ratio should be 5:1. When combining organic chelated calcium and magnesium, the absorption and utilization is greatly improved. My favorite form of calcium and magnesium is the citrate form, which is highly absorbable.

The easiest test for checking this is called the Calcium/Mg Cuff Test. This is a good test because calcium and magnesium are necessary for muscle relaxation. If you experience frequent muscle cramps or charlie horse of any kind, then you don't even need to do this test, you can be assured that your body has insufficient calcium/magnesium.

How to test:
Place a Blood Pressure cuff around the calf muscle, pump it up slowly and note when pressure cramping occurs. If the muscle begins to become painful and cramp before 160 mm of pressure, your calcium/magnesium ratio is out of balance and should be supplemented. Ideal pressure for this test is 220mm.

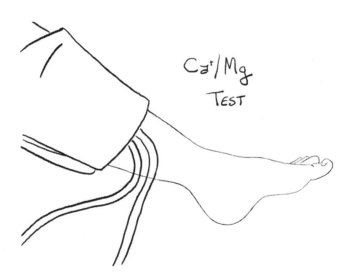

Ca⁺/Mg
TEST

12 - DIGESTIVE DOMINOS

ELEMENT—EARTH

*We Romans cram and poison ourselves with food and a succession of courses at a banquet. Sweet, sour, heavy, dainty, presented pell-mell in everyday vulgar profusion, confounding a man's palate and confusing his stomach with a detestable mixture of flavors, odors, and substances in which the true values are lost and the unique qualities disappear. Rather the Greeks know better—with grilled fish at the edge of the sea, vegetables so fresh and divinely clean, water directly from the spring—all diffusing within us the secret salt of the earth, and rain of heaven. All sick men should taste on their lips the small portions of this fresh simplicity. —*Hadrian

Amy is a 35-year-old patient of mine. Years ago, while in college, she developed poor digestion. At first she described it as a minor annoyance, but as time progressed she found herself with more and more constipation and with increasing levels of discomfort in her abdomen.

As an attempted solution, she began taking over-the-counter laxatives. After years of daily laxative use, she started seeing undigested food in her stools and began getting daily acid reflux. Bothered by this, she went to a gastroenterologist who suggested an antacid called Nexium to lessen the effects of the "heartburn" along with a colonoscopy. The colonoscopy showed several polyps but was otherwise normal. She took her doctor's advice and began the antacid medication.

Over the next six months she felt new symptoms coming to the surface. She developed anxiety, gained 20 pounds, started getting seasonal allergies and had low energy in the mornings. To combat these new symptoms she used coffee for energy and Valium to alleviate the anxiety. If she would drink too much coffee it would increase her anxiety, too little wouldn't provide enough energy. She felt her health was a mess.

Then came her first major breaking point: a chronic productive cough developed in which she expelled gobs of mucus. Becoming desperate for a solution, she sought out another doctor who performed an extensive medical physical, took blood, and performed X-rays of her lungs. The only abnormality found was high cholesterol. In addition to her laxatives, antacid, and Valium, this doctor added a steroid inhaler and cholesterol medication to her regimen.

She described the addition of these drugs as the second tipping point in her health. Soon after taking them, her blood pressure shot up 30 points.

Her final breaking point was the onset of daily, intense, and debilitating migraines. She finally came to the realization that she had to go outside the traditional medical system. It was the migraines that originally brought her to me in her search for new approach to her health.

Here's Amy's success story:

Amy regained full digestive capacity, lost weight, normalized her blood pressure, got off the medications and got her life back. The methods I used to cure her digestive ailments are carefully described in this chapter.

Amy's story is all too common in America today. America's declining health is linked to our weakened digestive capabilities. The obvious next step after consuming the right food is being able to absorb it. The inside of our digestion is actually considered the outside of our bodies. Until we absorb it, it's not ours...so after consuming good food, the final step of the Earth Element is absorbing the food. Hippocrates said, "All disease begins in the gut." He believed when digestion weakens, it's the number one cause of stress and disease in the body. As certain evidence of America's digestive strains, Americans purchase 300 million over the counter digestive relief drugs.

Many of us don't realize that good digestion is at the core of our health. We don't associate arthritis, skin conditions, joint pain, lowered immune system, allergies, autoimmune disease, weight gain, lowered fertility and many other symptoms to our poorly functioning bowels. Without proper digestion, a happy and healthy life is impossible. Joseph Conrad said it best, "The joy of life depends on a sound stomach whereas bad digestion inclines one to skepticism, incredulity, breeds black fancies, and thoughts of death."

Any health protocol that doesn't address and fix digestion is doomed to fail. Without proper digestive capacity there is no nutritional utilization in the body, making any diet, medication, or health system ineffective. On the other hand, even small improvements to the digestive system create significant improvements to the rest of the body. Regardless of your condition or health level, optimizing your digestion is an integral part of the answer. The WBH formula plainly lays out the solution to reconditioning your digestive dominoes.

I3 - STOMACH DOMINO

ELEMENT—EARTH

REMOVE: Antacids, Hiatal Hernia
ADD IN: Stomach Juices

I've loved dominoes ever since I was a kid. Not the game, but stacking them into a intricate long rows traversing tables, chairs and books throughout my room. The delight of pushing the first one and watching the natural progression of the remainder fall one after another brought a sense of satisfaction and joy because it perfectly complied with a natural order. If you could see inside your digestion, it would reveal the same natural order.

As you chew and break down food, the enzymes in your saliva prep the food for the acid bath that is your stomach. This in turn activates the liver, gallbladder and pancreas, also prepping the small intestines to absorb the nutrition for use in the body. After absorption, it passes into the colon that eventually eliminates the waste. If any of the dominoes don't activate, the remainder are doomed for failure. To correct digestion we must make sure each stage, each domino, is activating properly.

The first domino in your digestive health is your stomach acid. Hippocrates knew this and would frequently prescribe apple cider vinegar for almost all health issues. He knew that if there were not enough stomach acid juices, the first domino, and therefore the most important, would not fall.

If you want to cure your acid reflux and most digestive issues, you must add more acid into your stomach. This is a completely new and baffling statement to many. I gained insight into this issue by reading Jonathan Wright's book *Why Stomach Acid is Good for You*. Using the stomach juice test (described later), thousands of people have gotten off antacids and regained their digestive capacity and therefore their health.

Dr. Wright's book covers the myriad issues associated with low stomach acid. He references a Gallup Poll showing that 44% of Americans suffer from acid reflux at least one time per month. That's 140 million people searching to cure their digestion woes.

He goes on to site, reference, and document with hard scientific data that too little stomach acid causes almost all of these acid reflux cases. At first this might seem preposterous. How can acid reflux be caused by too little acid? The explanation is simple.

Digestion starts in the stomach. When food enters the acid bath in your stomach, it gyrates, pulses, and flexes. In short, it moves a lot like a washing machine. Essentially, the stomach is a churning acid bath. This turns the food into chyme before it enters the small intestine.

A normal stomach's pH should be around 2 (highly acidic). Amazingly, this pH level is more acidic than battery acid. It can burn through metal. Fortunately, the stomach has a lining that protects against its own acid. The stronger the acid, the more minimal the gyration time to break down the food into manageable proportions for the small intestine to absorb.

As food travels down the esophagus, it goes through a one way valve called the lower esophageal sphincter (LES). It closes tight, and prevents acid from splashing up into the esophagus. The esophagus doesn't have a lining like the stomach. If acid gets up in there, it burns painfully.

If there is not enough acid, the stomach has to shake around longer. This extended churning action creates back pressure on the esophageal sphincter (LES). This allows stomach contents, acid and all, to come back up the lower esophagus. Heartburn, reflux, or GERD is not actually burning of the stomach, but burning of the lower part of the esophagus.

The stomach does not want to release food until its stage of digestion is complete. The harder food is to digest, the longer it sits there as the stomach keeps churning away to try and break it down. Do you hear about people getting heartburn after a salad and soup? No. It's always after a Big Mac and large fries, or pizza and wings. Why? Because it's hard to digest. The body does everything it can, but when the stomach is slow in breaking down the food, acid reflex is the consequence of the excessive back pressure on the esophageal valve.

So, how do we get the dominoes to fall the other way towards healthy digestion? Should we block the acid and digestive capacity we have left? Or do we add to it?

Initially, antacids take the burn away. It's not because they heal it, but rather, they buffer and block the acid temporarily. Going the acid reflux medication route takes the pain away briefly, but it doesn't get to the root cause of the problem. Only the symptom is removed. The problem is still present and worsening. Antacids prevent full breakdown of food in the stomach. The partially digested food initiates the domino rows of disease. The long-term health effect of blocking acid is addictive and devastating.

This is exactly how it happened to Amy. This is exactly how it's happening to millions of Americans right now. In due course, antacids, like all drugs, make the condition worse, even though the reasoning behind cribing it is to make you feel better. It's close to the test lie ever told, and no one in the pharmaceutical industry will tell you the truth because they'll get fired.

Studies show that stomach acid and juices are highest during our teenage years. This is why your 15-year-old kid crushes an entire pizza with no problem whatsoever. Their large amounts of stomach juice break down even the most difficult foods.

As we age, our stomach acid and digestive capacity goes down and when we start to get symptoms of low acid most of us take medications to block the rest of it. Wouldn't it make sense to stop the decline of stomach acid instead? I've successfully treated thousands of people with acid reflux, indigestion, GERD, irritable bowel, constipation, and loose stools by increasing the acid in their stomach.

The acid bath consists of hydrochloric acid (HCL), pepsin, and shortly after, pancreatic enzymes. This concoction breaks down the protein we eat into amino acids. Amino acids are the necessary building blocks of DNA, muscle tissue, and neurotransmitters. The stomach juice concoction also breaks up and adsorbs minerals and many vitamins. Without proper digestion of protein, minerals, and vitamins, cellular function fades and long-term recovery from stress becomes impossible.

WBH APPROACH

When people come into my office actively complaining of acid reflux or heartburn, I immediately give them a few tablets of concentrated stomach juice (Hydrochloric acid, pepsin, and pancreatic enzymes), and wait 20 minutes. I try not to tell them what I'm giving them, because it's a tough sell when you tell someone with acid reflux that you want to give them more acid. After 20 minutes I ask them how they're doing and almost always they will tell me that the burning has subsided. Then, to their amazement, I tell them that I just gave them acid.

Seems backwards if you are not well-versed in true health, sort of like how eating fat can help you lose weight. The fact is that consuming more acid will fully complete your stomach digestion, therefore eliminating the symptoms of poor digestion and acid reflux. Below are a few test to know if you need to supplement stomach juices.

THE STOMACH PALPATION TEST

The stomach and pancreas tenderize and swell when stressed. By palpating along the lower edge of your left rib cage and the soft tissue located below there, you'll perceive the inflammation status of your stomach and pancreas. If this area is tender, you can be assured that your stomach juice and pancreatic enzyme production is insufficient. If this is tender and you have some of the symptoms listed below, then you should perform the stomach juice test.

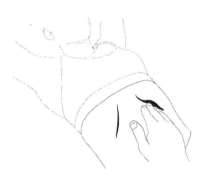

SYMPTOMS OF LOW STOMACH JUICE

- Need for over the counter (OTC) antacids (Prilosec, Tums, Zantac, etc.)
- Need for OTC laxatives
- History of intestinal parasites
- Food allergies
- IBS/ IBD / colitis
- Celiac disease
- Upper GI discomfort - GERD, indigestion
- Gastric ulcers
- Duodenal ulcers
- Stomach upset after eating meat protein
- Stomach churns / burns when empty
- Eating or drinking solves stomach pain
- Eating or drinking worsens stomach pain
- Diagnosed with reflux or GERD

THE STOMACH JUICE TEST

Performing this simple test on yourself can give you marvelous insight into your own stomach condition. The next time you have stomach symptoms do this: Take two tablets of concentrated stomach juices with every meal for one week. One of three things will happen:

1). It's going to help. You will feel better and the issue will go away. If you need still more stomach juice you will be noticeably better, you might just feel an increase in energy or less heaviness in your digestion. You now have performed an experiment on your own body and proven to yourself that you have insufficient stomach acid and juices to digest the foods you're eating.

2). It's going to make you worse. The acid reflux, heartburn or chest pain will increase. If this happens you have a hiatal hernia. A hiatal hernia is when your stomach is too high up into your chest and the one-way valve (lower esophageal sphincter) that's supposed to keep all the juices in the stomach is stuck open. This allows food and acid to come back up and give you discomfort. If this is the case the stomach needs to be actively pulled down under the hiatus. While sometimes you can do this to yourself, usually it requires someone to help you. If having someone helping you: Have them place their fingers of both hands at the bottom of your sternum palpating down underneath the bottom rib on the left side two inches from the sternum. This is where the bottom your stomach is located. Have them push inward and downward with about 10 lbs of pressure. Have them hold this for 2 minutes while you the patient breathe deeply from the stomach. Often a noticeable release will be felt as the stomach returns to where it should be. Doing this is powerful and can often fix a hiatal hernia in a few sessions.

3). Nothing changes. Your symptoms are most likely not caused by low stomach acid.

Why has no one ever told you this before? Is it because the antacid business is making $10 billion per year? No, it can't be that...Sadly, the considerable amount of marketing money spent on promoting this industry serves only to confuse the issue.
Concentrated stomach juice (Hcl and enzymes) is cheap and you can fix your own hiatal hernia for free. For more information on how to fix a hiatal hernia, see Appendix D explaining this procedure. Don't Google this. You'll only complicate the matter and confuse yourself even more until you fully learn the WBH formula.

As the fully digested acid soup (chyme) leaves your stomach it signals your liver and pancreas to release bile, bicarbonate, and enzymes, so on we go to the second domino.

14- LIVER AND GALLBLADDER DOMINO

ELEMENT—EARTH

REMOVE: Alcohol, processed vegetable oils
ADD IN: Liver support, liver flushes

The next step of digestion involves the production of bile from the liver and released by the gallbladder. Bile is a dark green fluid consisting of water, bile salts, bilirubin, and other salts. It's alkaline with a pH of 9. Manufactured by the liver and stored in the gallbladder, it is absolutely necessary for digestion of fats.

The liver is the hardest working, most complex, and heaviest organ in the body, and continuously produces 1-2 liters of bile every day. The gallbladder is a sac which has the sole purpose to store and pump bile when fats are consumed. The complexity of this may give us perspective on the cruciality of fat breakdown to the body. (Side note: Never surgically remove your gallbladder unless it's necrotic. If your doctor recommends it for any other reason, refuse and give him or her a copy of this book.)

Bile's critical function is to help neutralize stomach acid and emulsify fat prior to the chyme entering the small intestine. In addition, it helps destroy any microbes that might have somehow survived the stomach's acid bath.

The liver has intra-hepatic duct work, which are thousands of channels for bile drainage. It's kind of like the plumbing system in your house, but way more complex and extensive. Normalized, free-flowing liver and bile are essential to digest fats, remove built-up cholesterol and hormones from your body, digest fat soluble vitamins, and allow enzymes to function. Additionally, the liver makes and removes 80% of the cholesterol in the body. With over 500 known functions, the liver is essential to the body's function and nothing works right if the liver and bile can't drain properly.

Are you beginning to get it? Let me put it to you in highly technical and scientific terminology: The liver is really freaking important and if it gets plugged, you're in trouble!

Healthy bile production and release is essential for human health. If bile production isn't sufficient, fats become rancid in the body, leading to severe breakdown in the intestines. These rancid fats act as powerful free radicals destroying cellular function throughout the body.

Overconsumption of sugar and processed foods are the number one cause of bile obstruction. Furthermore, bad fats and oils from processed foods clog liver drainage. The next time you go to movies and order popcorn with partially hydrogenated soybean oil on it (butter), remember this: it's going to take over six months to process through your liver.

Because all of us love movie popcorn and sugar and the 82,000 other chemicals in our world, virtually every unhealthy adult in America suffers from insufficient bile production. Even a small decrease over time will increase the likelihood of disease. When this bile becomes thick it can't flow and eventually turns to sludge and, finally, stones. Most people have hundreds, even thousands of these thick sludge-like pebbles in their liver and gallbladder blocking bile drainage.

I vividly remember examining a gall bladder packed with stones in graduate-level anatomy class. They were rocks. The stones were plugs for all intents and purposes, blocking all possible bile drainage. It wasn't hard to figure out why this particular human corpse was laying in front of me for dissection.

Here are some reasons for the importance of optimal liver function:

- It processes sugar that you eat, converting it to usable energy when needed
- It converts thyroid hormone from inactive to an active form
- It creates bile for fat digestion
- It removes hormones from the body—most especially estrogen and epinephrine
- It detoxifies toxins and poisons from the body (including sugar)
- It responds and reduces free-radical damage and inflammation
- It has strong anti-mutagenic (cancer) properties

Ancient Ayurvedic medicine has known the importance and the properties of the liver and bile for thousands of years. Many of the diseases of modern culture are created from the toxemia created by poor liver drainage. The point of this explanation is this: As part of the WBH formula we need to clear the plumbing of your liver and gallbladder as an essential step in healing.

Four things must be done to keep the plumbing in the liver clear and bile production high:

1. Avoid processed fats (all processed vegetable oils—soybean, canola, Crisco, etc.)

2. Remove all sugar, alcohol and processed foods from the diet.

3. Consume foods and supplements that help with liver drainage. This includes beets, beet leaves, liver and all vegetables. For supplements I suggest a product called Liver/GB Drainage which helps with the free flow of bile.

4. Perform regular liver flushes. This should be performed once during the last week of the 21 day reset, then quarterly (4 times per year afterwards). The step-by-step process for performing the liver flush is outlined in Appendix E.

Liver flush! Delightful!

As gross as it sounds, flushing out accumulated sludge, cholesterol, bile, and stones from your liver is a necessity if you want to achieve vibrant health. For well-researched information, read the book *The Amazing Liver Flush*. Depending on the severity of the case, it can take many rounds of liver flushes and extended liver supplementation for full bile production recovery. Once the liver blockages are gone the liver has the ability to heal and miraculously regenerate. Its regenerative qualities are substantially greater than any other organ in the body. This is another testament to the importance of a healthy liver. Once it's improved, your body can process the necessary high fat diet needed for whole body health.

SYMPTOMS OF POOR LIVER AND BILE PRODUCTION

∘ Hard potbelly with little body fat
∘ Craving for fatty, fried, and sour foods

- Joint degeneration and arthritic
- Yellowing of the whites of the eyes
- Morning bloodshot eyes
- Frequent skin rashes, hives, and/or itch
- Bouts of eczema and/or psoriasis
- Little red dots on skin
- Bloating after eating ✓
- Hemorrhoids and/or itchy anus
- Sensitivities to perfumes/chemicals
- Basel, migraine and/or TMJ headaches
- Tendency for bruising
- High cholesterol
- High triglycerides
- Varicose or spider veins
- Urine darker and more odorous in morning
- Noticeable white coated tongue
- Overheating of body, especially hot feet at night
- Foot soles peeling
- Low morning appetite or skip breakfast altogether
- Chronic daily alcohol consumer
- Digestion upset upon eating fat
- Gallbladder pains and/or light-colored stools
- Excessive burping or belching after eating
- Acid reflux after eating fatty foods
- Reoccurring bouts of constipation ✓
- Wake-up between 1-3 am ✓
- Stiffness and pain between shoulder blades
- Indiscriminate pressure just under right rib cage
- Roll of fat below ribs, seen mostly in women

Are you seeing some symptoms that you recognize?

Most of us do. It's hard to live in this toxic world and not get a backed up liver. Let these symptoms motivate you to reduce the stress on your liver and elevate you to a happier life.

THE GALLBLADDER PALPATION TEST

A good test, similar to the palpation of the stomach, is the palpation of the liver for tenderness. This is also called Murphy's Sign. It's better if you can get someone else to do this to you as it's difficult to perform on your own. Have someone push just below your right rib cage right where your gall bladder is located. While you breathe out, have them place about 10 pounds of pressure right over your gallbladder. If it is full, inflamed and needs drainage, the pain will let you know immediately.

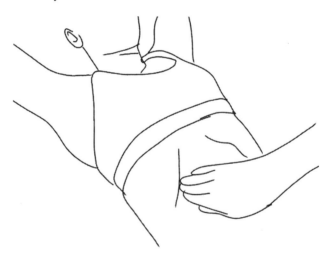

THE LIVER BODY TYPE

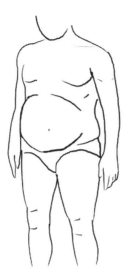

    Men especially, but also women, develop a larger belly out of proportion with the rest of the fat on their body. This is a clear indication of liver and bile dysfunction.

    The solutions to a backed-up liver are going to take time. Be sure to follow the above steps if you have the body type, the symptoms and the palpation test is tender. Eat the right diet, take the supplements, avoid the bad fats and do the liver flushes. Once your liver is right, then the third domino can fall—small intestine absorption.

15 - SMALL INTESTINE DOMINO

ELEMENT—EARTH

REMOVE: Foods which lack enzymes, food
    allergens, leaky gut.
ADD IN: Enzymes, allergy elimination technique

The third domino in the digestion process is the small intestine. By the time food gets to this point, it has turned into chyme. The stomach should have broken all the protein bonds, the liver should have emulsified all the fat and alkalized the chyme, and now it's ready for absorption. The small intestine utilizes enzymes to extract valuable nutrition. Of course, the assumption is that the food you ate contained enzymes, or you still had enzymes left in your reserves. Let me explain:

Pasteurization, canning, or cooking food over 115 degrees destroys enzymes. In short, processed food is 'dead' food, because it's devoid of enzymes. If dead food is consumed, our body uses its enzyme reserves to aid with digestion. The more enzymes we use up in our reserves, the quicker we age and the closer we get to a health crisis. This crucial concept must be understood. Dr. Francis M. Pottenger, Jr.'s seminal research documented this.

The story of Dr. Pottenger and his cats is a fascinating foray into the epigenetic effects of diet and the importance of enzymes. Dr. Pottenger is to me the godfather of epigenetics. Epigenticis is the concept that our genetics are not set at birth but rather determined by how we live. Dr. Pottenger, along with Dr. Price, showed us that epigenetics is actually generational health. He conducted his research with his cats, showing how diet could change and reverse gene expression; not only in their life, but in the generations of kittens that followed. But the real reason I am telling his story is digestive enzymes.

POTTENGER'S CATS

In 1930, Dr. Pottenger began a study with the initial intent of finding a standardized dose of adrenal supplementation in cats. Cats donated by a local shelter underwent surgery to remove their adrenal glands. After surgery he supplemented them with adrenal extracts in order to find a standardized dose with the hope of extrapolating his findings to human tuberculosis patients.

While working with these cats, he fed them the same cooked meat, pasteurized milk, and cod liver oil as the patients from his sanatorium ate. However, kitchen staff complaints of food shortage necessitated ordering food for the cats from a local meat packing plant and farm that supplied it as raw scraps of organ meat, raw milk and bone. At this point, the research took quite an interesting turn.

He noticed that not only did more cats eating the raw food better survive from their adrenalectomy, but the felines looked healthier and seemed happier than the ones he continued to feed the usual cooked food from the sanatorium's kitchen.

The difference between the two groups of cats was profound: "Within a very short time the cats in the pens [fed raw meat] survived the operations...appeared to be in better health, and the kittens born were vigorous," he wrote. "The contrast in apparent health between the

157

cats in the pens fed on raw-meat scraps and those fed on the cooked-meat scraps was startling."77

With these observations, he changed the course of his experiment to studying the effects of raw food on multiple generations of cats. By using animals with shorter generational timeframes and similar digestive and neurological chemistry as humans, he was able to forecast how dietary decisions affect future generations on humans. This experiment was the first ever conceived that studied the intricately woven relationship of multi-generational gene expression, enzymes, and diet. What he found was that cats fed the raw diet had:

○ Full pregnancies with an average of 5 kittens
○ No problems birthing or nursing
○ Strong immune systems
○ Broad faces, normal dental arches, regular teeth, healthy bone structure

As Dr. Pottenger put it: "Their organic development was complete and functioning normal." In other words, they were healthy, beautiful, and fully expressing their genetic potential in life. He in turn studied the next three generations, and found the case to be the same with each subsequent litter. They too were healthy and fully expressing life.

Cats fed the cooked (less or no enzymes) diet:
○ Lack of symmetry in skeletal structures
○ Unable to carry to full term pregnancy
○ Labored and difficult births, often ending in mortality
○ Smaller litters
○ Frequent failures to nurse with insufficient lactation

The subsequent two generations fed the cooked diet:
- Rare, and problematic pregnancies
- Females: irritable, often biting and scratching.
- Males: passive, didn't pursue mates or copulation.
- Major health problems, including skin lesions, skeletal deformation, and a variety of dental conditions such as irregular spacing and/or lack of teeth.

After the third generation he could no longer continue with the experiment because pregnancy and birth rates had dropped almost to zero.

A couple of conclusions:

1. Cats on a diet of cooked food (less enzymes), were less healthy and passed down their poor health to their children over three generations, with each generation becoming less healthy and fertile than the previous until the generational line perished.

2. Something essential for health was being lost in food during processing and cooking. It would be discovered later that the something lost was the enzymes (the life of food). Enzymes are heat sensitive and at 115 degrees (Fahrenheit) they are destroyed.

Dr. Pottenger didn't stop here. His insatiable curiosity drove him to the next level of the study. He wondered whether he could reverse the condition of the sick felines by feeding them the diet of the healthy cats. So, he changed the diet of the unhealthy cats from the cooked meats to the raw food that he was feeding the healthy cats. To his delight, he found that he reactivated healthy characteristics for future generations, and almost unbelievably each subsequent generation of cats born regained their health. However it took four generations to get to the optimal feline health that had been lost during the previous three generations.

As often stated, the sins of the fathers will be visited upon their sons. How would our society function if our overriding decisions were based on the Native American principle that we must choose our actions according to how they will affect the next seven generations? How would our own decisions change if we knew the junk food we ate directly hurt our children?

While Dr. Pottenger never "claimed" that the health of cats can be exactly compared to that of humans, through empirical observation, the similarities between what he found and what's happening to the American population are uncannily similar.

ENZYMES IN AMERICA

Enzymes are the "life" of food. Want to see an enzyme at work? Leave fruit out on the counter and watch it ripen. Enzymes break down food. Ever leave a Big Mac, large fries, and a Coke out on the counter from our favorite purveyor of fine junk foods? You're going to sit there for years watching, because it won't rot. Why? No enzymes. So what happens to what my father calls a "chlorine-bleached, antibiotic-laced, hormone-filled, toxic abomination called a Happy Meal" when we eat it?

When an alligator captures its food in the wild it drowns it, then lets it go for several days to weeks before eating it. Why? It innately knows that enzymes are breaking down the meat and making it more digestible. We humans know this innately too. Want a great steak, go eat a dry-aged one. The steak is hung up and aged for weeks, allowing enzymes to work their magic. This makes the meat tender, delicious, and easily digestible.

For the last 150 years, since the time of Louis Pasteur, the diet of America has changed in a way

160

designed to destroy enzymes. It turns out that when we heat and pasteurize food, we kill the enzymes along with the bacteria. Enzymes are how the food breaks down but also the same mechanism as how food spoils. Thus incentivizing food manufacturers to kill all the enzymes.

This starts on an agricultural level with the use of insecticides. Insecticides work by shutting down the enzyme system of bugs. These same insecticides were effectively used in World War I nerve gas. So you won't be surprised to learn that the same company that produced nerve gas and Agent Orange also produces modern day insecticides—Monsanto.[78] Then, to further stop spoilage, food manufacturers use radon gas and carbon monoxide to kill any enzymes still alive in produce. Non-produce is pasteurized, processed, and canned to kill off all the enzymes. When enzyme life in food ceases to exist, our own metabolic enzymes decrease to try to compensate for the dead indigestible food in our guts. Dr. Royal Lee started the first whole food nutritional supplement company called Standard Process. He said, "Enzymes are the most important unit in the human body, because every chemical change that takes place involves the activity of enzymes. Without enzyme activity there is no life. No plant or animal can live without the activity of its enzymes."

We are approaching the third and fourth generation of Americans that have eaten a low-enzyme diet and with it we're finding all the same symptoms that Dr. Pottenger found with his cats. Infertility rates are high and increasing, 90% of Americans' teeth rot, over 50% of our children need braces, mood is affected, and joy is disappearing. According to the World Health Organization, 350 million adults suffer from depression and it's the leading cause of disability.

We're born with a limited amount of enzymes, kind of like how a woman is born with only so many eggs. It's all we get. If we run out due to eating too many Happy Meals, it's impossible for the human body to catalyze the millions of required daily chemical actions—which means we get sick.

TYPES OF ENZYMES

There are thousands of varieties of metabolic enzymes including delta desaturase, superoxide dismutase, glutathione peroxidase, and many more required for nutrient conversion, liver function, and cellular expression. Our digestive process alone necessitates 22 separate enzymes including pancreatin, pepsin and trypsin. Digestive enzymes are supposed to be in our foods, these include:

- Amylase, to break down starch
- Protease, to break down protein
- Lipase, to break down fat
- Cellulase, to break down fiber
- Lactase, to break down dairy
- Sucrase, to break down sugar
- Maltase, to break down grains

According to the Food Renegade blog, "Your body needs [enzymes] to properly digest, absorb, and make full use of your food. As you age, your body's supply of enzymes decreases. This has caused many scientists to hypothesize that if you could guard against enzyme depletion, you could live a longer, healthier life." That reminds me of the old Chinese proverb that states, "A man can only eat so many grains of rice in his life, with the last one he dies."

Studies show that by the time we're 70 years old we have 20% of the enzymes we had when we were 20.[79] Our digestion is basically a bag full of enzymes and bacteria. When we eat raw food such as raw milk, meat cooked rare, and fermented vegetables that have not been radiated or gassed, no metabolic enzymes are required for digestion. They literally digest themselves. Everything needed for proper digestion is contained within the food!

Constant gas, belching, bloating, and discomfort in the abdomen are the most noticeable symptoms that your metabolic tank of enzymes is on low. Dr. William Kelly, a holistic physician who successfully treated cancer patients, used to say that gas was the best warning system for cancer. He would give people pancreatic enzymes and if they felt better and their gas went away, it would indicate that their bodies were at risk for cancer. His next step would be to dose pancreatic enzymes at high volumes to help the body break down the cancer.

The most obvious symptom that your digestive enzymes are low is gas. The food is not fully breaking down and therefore it's producing gas. Gas is not normal. Just because it has always been normal to you or in your house, it is a strong indication of a problem.

Interestingly enough, the smell of our gas is very telling as to which enzyme systems are low. If that gas is extremely foul smelling, it's probably protein that is putrefying and creating that noxious, room-clearing stink that many people blame on the dog. If the gas is produced by carbohydrates, the smell won't be nearly as bad, but it still reveals a serious enzyme deficiency. Any deficiency of enzymes allows food to rot inside us creating toxemia and then illness. The book *Toxemia Explained* says it like this: "Every so-called disease is a crisis of toxemia, which means that toxin has accumulated in the blood above the toleration point... The crisis, the so-called disease—call it cold, flu, pneumonia, headache, or typhoid fever—is a vicarious elimination. Nature is endeavoring to rid the body of toxins."

What is your Digestive Enzyme Level?

- Ideal = No digestive complaints
- Stage 1 = Mild gas, inconsistent stool quality and quantity
- Stage 2 = Moderate gas, occasional burping, non-consistent stool quality and quantity
- Stage 3 = Offending gas, frequent burping, abdominal pain, OTC digestive aids, constipation and/or regular diarrhea

So, back to the small intestine domino...

Once the food enters the small intestine there are millions of microvilli (little fingers) that "absorb" all the nutrition and calories, carry them to your transport system known as your blood, which delivers them to each cell of the body. The efficient design of the microvilli ability to increase absorption is so great that you could stretch their surface space to the size of a tennis court.

When food is not fully digested because of lack of enzymes, the body produces mucus to coat and protect the microvilli from damage as the food moves through the intestines. This is a normal process...until it's no longer normal. It's no longer normal when the mucus backs up throughout your entire body. It's impossible to eat processed, enzyme-less food like McDonald's burgers and not have accumulation of undigested food and mucus in your intestines.

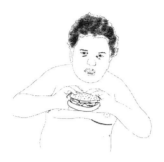

I know I'm harping on McDonald's a lot, but seriously does anyone still eat there? Trust me, no matter how much they spend on their marketing to brainwash us that "I'm lovin' it" when we think of their golden arches, the McDonald's corporation doesn't love us. If they did, they would pick up the medical bill for the collective damage they have done to global health.

Arnold Ehret's classic book *Mucus-less Diet Healing System* goes into depth about the necessity to use enzyme-rich raw foods to remove the collected mucus in the body. Without its removal, autointoxication and eventually disease is the only possible outcome.

As mucus accumulates in the small intestine and large intestine, it turns into a hardened version known as mucoid plaque. Mucoid plaque is just as it sounds: it's a hardened, blackened mass of mucous providing haven for the bad bacteria, fungus, candida, viruses and parasites that love it.

The point of this entire chapter is that enzyme supplementation is essential for regaining health, digesting the undigested food in your gut, and refilling your metabolic enzyme bank account. Enzymes in food are insufficient to have a chance at catching up. There

many plant-based broad spectrum enzymes on the
market. Here is my recommendation: if you are in good
health (perfect digestion, no gas, no health issues
whatsoever), take one tablet of enzymes any time you
eat a meal that is not raw food. If you are not healthy,
take three enzymes with every meal. Do this until all
bloating, gas and health issues are gone and then go back
to only taking enzymes with only cooked food. For the
purpose of the 21 day reset, make sure you're taking nine
enzyme tablets per day. If you have a serious disease,
double it to 18 tablets per day. For many, it can easily
take up to six months of enzyme supplementation to get
caught up with the undigested food in your intestines.

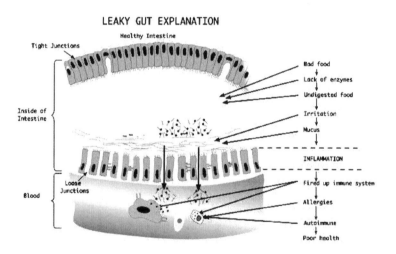

LEAKY SMALL INTESTINE

As you can see from the illustration, the
accumulation of mucus creates inflammation and
damage to intestinal walls. It's inevitable that the longer
you eat an enzyme-deficient diet the quicker and more
likely you or future generations will reach a tipping
point. Leaky gut is that tipping point. Medical doctors

call it intestinal permeability or intestinal hyper-permeability.

A lack of enzymes directly result in mucoid plaque build up. Too much mucus fills up the intestine, creating inflammation in the intestinal walls. Chronic inflammation causes microscopic holes and tears to appear, making the intestinal walls porous.

The tight junctions of the small intestine's cells become weakened and this allows rotten and undigested particles of food, microbes, and toxins to leak into the blood stream. The immune system views the undigested food as a foreign invader, which it then attacks.

All five of the top over-the-counter drugs used in America are associated with leaky gut. Ignoring symptoms of leaky gut is akin to ignoring your car's low oil light or smashing it because the red color bothers you.

Top five OTC medications:
1. Antihistamines/cough/cold medications (771m units)
2. Analgesics, or pain medications (443m)
3. Anti-gas products, or antacid medications (173m)
4. Laxatives (114m)
5. Diarrhea medications (22m)

SYMPTOMS OF LEAKY GUT

- Allergies (both food and environmental)
- Autoimmune disease
- Arthritis
- Thyroid disease
- Malabsorption
- Inflammation anywhere in the body
- Heartburn

- Belching
- Bloating and gas
- Constipation
- Loose bowels
- Chronic pain such as fibromyalgia
- Irritability, anxiety, depression, cognitive deficits, brain fog
- Chronic diseases such as diabetes, cancer, heart disease, arthritis

The strongest stressor on a body, one that *always* results in final failure, is the compromise of the barrier between the gut and the blood. The loss of this barrier means rapid changes need to be made or disease is inevitable. The dominoes can be set up to fall in the wrong direction as well.

Allergies kick in as soon as the gut becomes leaky. This is usually when people find they are unable to eat gluten, dairy or nightshades, and get seasonal allergies and a hundred other food sensitivities. If allergies go long enough they turn into autoimmune disease.

Many people don't know that they have food allergies and possibly autoimmune disease. All they know is that they don't feel good most of the time. As time goes on, they get diagnosed with conditions such as celiac, mood disorders, Hashimoto's disease, developmental disorders, cancer, heart disease, Alzheimer's, obesity, chronic fatigue, IBS, fibromyalgia and many others. This is the most common mechanism for why people get sick.

Out of desperation, many of these people beg their doctor to test them for gluten sensitivity, food allergies, or autoimmune disease. Unfortunately, most people don't get a diagnosis until they ask their doctor for it, and most doctors don't know how to diagnose it. The

American Autoimmune Disease Association did a survey of physicians and found only 12% of physicians felt they had adequate training about autoimmune disease and only 4% felt comfortable diagnosing it.

As a result, most don't get the proper diagnosis early enough because autoimmune disease starts years before serious symptoms or disease become obvious. This period between when we start getting sensitive and get sick is called the Prodromal Period. It is the first stage of disease, and the period in which you just feel bad.

Standard allergy testing does little to help people. This is because many food allergies have multiple peptides (protein molecules) yet often they test just one or two. Wheat, for example, has 62 different peptides that you can become allergic to. When doctors test for gluten sensitivity they usually only test the most common allergenic peptide called the Alpha Glidden Peptide. If you are allergic to any of the other 61 peptides your doctor will tell you that you are not allergic to gluten. Whoops, and it's the same for many different foods and many autoimmune conditions. The testing is expensive and highly inaccurate.

The National Institutes of Health tells us that 50% of Americans suffer from allergies and 24 million people have been diagnosed with autoimmune disease. NIH estimates that only one in three people with autoimmune disease is actually diagnosed. This means that there are at least 75 million undiagnosed people in our country with autoimmune disease, leaky gut, food allergies, and an enzyme deficiency.

FIXING LEAKY GUT

The key to fixing leaky gut begins with first eating real food and eliminating all carbohydrates. This means all grains and dairy. Then, by increasing digestive juices (stomach, liver, and enzymes) we will stop the creation of inflammation and mucus buildup caused by undigested food in the intestines.

If, after 21 days of living like this, your health dramatically improves, you lose weight, your energy goes up, and you become a happier person, then you know that food and digestion is part of your issue. Then, if you like, over the next two months, slowly reintroduce the foods and watch for a return of symptoms. If any symptoms arise with a certain food, simply eliminate it from your diet. It can take years to fully heal leaky gut. Some with very damaged guts are going to need almost perfect diets for several years to maintain wellness. Finally, to fully address allergies, one should also incorporate Kinesiology Muscle Testing and Allergy Elimination Techniques.

MUSCLE TESTING FOR ALLERGIES

A highly effective approach for determining food allergies is muscle testing. Muscle testing is the single best method for testing food sensitivity. This is done by simply holding a food and having someone muscle test you for weakness. Through this method, one can get immediate biofeedback if the food is shutting down your body. Muscle testing works energetically. The body, through touch or taste, senses the allergy and diverts nerve energy away from the muscles and toward the immune system, resulting in a 'weak' muscle. In my office, we muscle test everyone for the primary allergies to wheat, gluten, corn, soy, nuts, rice, nightshades, milk,

170

and shellfish. Those that shut off muscle strength tell us with 100% accuracy that they are stressors and should be avoided.

While avoidance of food is very beneficial, people often run into the problem that many foods are hidden. Gluten, for example, is in powdered eggs, soy sauce, candy, and a thousand other items. Corn is in almost all processed foods, in toiletries, and many medications. This makes avoidance difficult. Each time someone is unknowingly exposed to allergies, their body diverts its energy to the immune system to handle the perceived invading army.

The solution to this issue is a technique called Allergy Elimination Technique. After one identifies and avoids foods/environmental allergies that weaken, then Allergy Elimination Technique should begin. Allergy elimination is a way of turning off the body's response to foods. While this concept of allergy elimination sounds impossible at first glance, it's incredibly effective at resetting the body's response systems.

Think of your allergies and body's response like this: You would not soon forget a burglar's face if you walked into your home and saw him stealing all your possessions. The burglar was created by low enzymes, leaky gut, and a fired-up immune system response. If you ever came home and saw the burglar again you would immediately go into emergency mode even if this person gave up crime and had no intention of stealing from you.

This is often what's happening in your body with food. Once a food sensitivity is recognized by your immune system the body is not going to forget it. However, there is a method we use that essentially wipes the memory of your body toward food allergies so your body is not constantly attacking itself. It's akin to turning off your immune system's computer and rebooting it. It's powerful and free, which is why you've

171

probably never heard of it before. It makes your body forget the criminal's face so the next time they arrive... no response.

By balancing someone's acupuncture meridians while they hold the allergen the automated immune response turns off. Let's say a stranger walked into your house, your dog started barking like crazy and you calmed the dog and told it everything was ok. The dog would think, "OK, if my master's cool with this guy then so am I," and the next time the new guy showed up the dog would probably lick them.

When our body energetically recognizes a foreign invader, our immune system starts barking. If we balance our acupuncture meridians while touching the allergen, the immune system says, "OK, if you're cool with this allergen then so am I." An explanation of how to muscle test and perform Allergy Elimination can be found in Appendix D. This technique was pioneered by a woman named Dr. Devi Nambudripad, and she writes extensively about it in her book *Say Goodbye to Illness.*

Read her book for a more complete explanation of the technique, the theory behind why it works so well, or many motivational patient stories. I have witnessed thousands of people's lives dramatically healed with the Allergy Elimination technique, and it is an essential step along the Whole Body Health path.

Finally, let's move on to the colon.

16 - COLON DOMINO

ELEMENT—EARTH

REMOVE: Antibiotics, foods that kill probiotics, candida, and fungus
ADD IN: Fermented foods and probiotics

The final domino of digestion is healthy colon function. The colon's function is simple and vital. It absorbs the remaining water and nutrients while converting digested food into feces. The actual miracle of the colon is the bacterial life forms residing within it. There are 400 to 700 billion bacteria living in your colon that are responsible for a healthy body and mind.

I was amazed when I first read the research that over 95% of serotonin (the feel-good hormone) is produced and used by the intestines. The digestive tract also produces over 30 other neurotransmitters including norepinephrine, melatonin, and dopamine. All this is made possible by the bacteria in our gut.

The human body has somewhere around 30-40 billion human cells, but has as much as 10-20 times as many bacteria. DNA expression depends on this bacteria. According to fossil records, bacteria was the first life-force on this planet. Therefore, in a way, bacteria are our ancestors, still dispensing wisdom from within our gut. We pass it on from generation to generation through healthy natural births, when our mother's vaginal canal coats us with her bacteria. This bacterial coating seeds within us as babies, providing us with countless gifts of all our previous generations, including imprinting our immune system with appropriately robust responses to disease. **Bacteria is our epigenetic birthright.** "We are literally losing our birthright," my M.D. father used to tell me. We receive our microbial baptism at birth as we are born through the birth canal. The increased use of C-sections is breaking the chain of generational microbes. Vaccines and antibiotics early in a child's life further diminishes our body's microbe biodiversity.

This is why using antibiotics to wage nuclear warfare on our gut biome will one day be looked upon as an insane period of medical history akin to bloodletting. Dr. Proctor, a professor of medicine at Stanford University School of Medicine puts it like this: "When you're looking in the mirror, what you're really looking at is 10 times more microbial cells than human cells" and "In almost every measure you can think of, we're more microbial than human." Martin Blaser, who directs the human micro-biome program at NY Langone Medical Center says: "As micro-biome organisms are lost, diseases have just skyrocketed." He lists diabetes, celiac, asthma, allergies, obesity, and developmental disorders as a direct consequence of loss of bacterial diversity within our gut.

THE WAR ON BACTERIA

As you continue to wrap your head around the concept of health and disease, you now realize that the terrain of your body is of the utmost importance. Like magnetic polarities, a healthy body repels disease. An unhealthy body attracts it.

This has always been the case. Take for example our species and its proliferation. The Earth's environment (terrain) is favorable to us and we thrive on it. The inhospitable terrain of the moon on the other hand, though quite interesting to visit on occasion, is not exactly prime real estate for human living.

Bacteria adapted to all of Earth. If you were provided with magical glasses that could make you see bacterial life in color, you would see rainbows upon rainbows of exploding color on every surface. They are everywhere, and have been so for billions of years before humans, and will continue for billions of more years, even if humans go extinct. They cannot be killed because they make Earth a living planet. In other words, if the bacteria are gone, all life on Earth is gone. The planet's terrain would be lifeless without them and you wouldn't be here.

By learning to encourage the proliferation of good bacteria, we can nourish our own gut community. The good ones compete for space with the unhealthy bacteria. My father used to tell me that "our bodies are like a stadium with 100 trillion seats and they all need to be filled. If they're not filled with the beneficial bacteria then they will be filled with destructive ones."

Bacteria, yeast, and fungus are everywhere. We cannot kill them off. So why would we try when the only result is resistant bacteria that develop into better equipped and stronger strains to take over unhealthy human bodies?

The best arrangement with bacteria is to follow the Golden Rule with them. Let's love them. They are our neighbors, our ancestors and our friends. They are offering their help by living in our guts. Why would we destroy the bacterial hand that feeds us?

We must engage in altruistic action with bacteria and exponentially create mutual well being. Our current tactic of waging all out nuclear warfare with them in the form of antibiotics has dangerously backfired. Our diplomatic relations veered off-course because we humans have lost sight of our symbiotic relationship with them.

More recently, scientists were surprised to learn that 90% of the fibers in the primary visceral nervous system and vagus nerves (heart, lung control) carry information from the gut to the brain, *not* from the brain to the gut. Think about what this means for our emotions, DNA expression, and our identity. In many ways our emotions, mood, and thoughts are determined by bacteria from our gut and not from our brain.

Researchers using gene profiling found that the absence of gut bacteria during infancy (C-section, vaccines, antibiotics, sterile home environment) permanently alters genes and signaling pathways involved in learning, memory, and motor control. Proper gut bacteria also help hundreds of your genes to express in a positive, disease-fighting manner.

In children, gut bacteria has shown to affect body weight for a lifetime. One study found babies with a high number of Bifido bacteria and low number of Staphylococcus appear to be protected from weight gain and obesity for life. Another study found that obese people that had 20% more bad bacteria and 90% less good bacteria than lean people.

Let's learn to love our little bacterial friends and drop the war with them. They are actually humanity's ally. Throw out the Purell, pitch the Lysol, play in the dirt, and kiss more people on the mouth. The more bacteria we swap the better. Without constant exposure to bacteria and microbes in food and soil, we do not have contact with the life form that is directly responsible for human happiness.

Having abundant, healthy bacteria makes it very difficult for the body to become ill. Without it, the body will literally attract infections. Rudolf Virchow, the German "Pope of Medicine" stated: **"If I could live** my life over again, I would devote it to proving that germs seek their natural habitat: diseased tissue, rather than being the cause of diseased tissue."

FACTORS IN THE DESTRUCTION OF BENEFICIAL BACTERIA

- Antibiotics
- Antibiotics given to the animals whose meat we eat
- Prescription and over the counter medications
- White sugar and white carbohydrates
- Carbonated drinks
- Antihistamines
- Chlorinated water
- Fluoridated water
- Coffee

SYMPTOMS OF COLON DYSFUNCTION

- Gas, bloating
  Lack of normal bowel movements (normal is brown, large, no pain or strain)
- Strain when having a bowel movement
- Cramping or pain with bowel movements
  Abdominal cramping or pain w/out bowel movement
- Undigested food evident in stool
- Bouts of diarrhea
- Stool: small and hard
- Stool: thin (pencil like)
- Stool: loose
- Stool: very foul smelling
- Gas: moderate to foul odor

I still remember in my first year of practice when I went to a church party. I was out of school, just started my practice, and was looking forward to get acquainted with my community. While at the party a woman asked me if I could possibly help her child with his chronic ear infections. She described how her 6-year-old son had been prescribed antibiotics 12 times in the last two years and yet he was still suffering from chronic infections. More recently her pediatrician advised a permanent low dose of antibiotics.

I couldn't believe it! A permanent dose of antibiotics? I asked her again to make sure. She confirmed that yes, her son was on a permanent low daily dose of antibiotics.

I told her that the first step was to rebuild her son's autoimmune system by stopping the antibiotics immediately. I explained to her the antibiotics were destroying the healthy bacteria in her child's system, which directly correlates with decreased immune system function. I advised her to stop feeding the child all sugar and diary immediately. I explained that refined sugar was toxic, and her son's body was using up precious minerals and vitamins to expel the sugar. I told her to replace drugs and antibiotics with echinacea and vitamin C and a probiotic supplements. Then I told her to get the child chiropractic adjustments to improve nerve flow and lymphatic drainage around the ears.

It turned out that her pediatrician was at the party and heard me describing this common sense approach to ear infections. He first asked me if I was an M.D., and when I told him I was not, he looked at me and told me my recommendations were wrong, that I was a quack, and recommended that the woman should avoid me.

I was flabbergasted. How did we get to this point in healthcare in which recommending a child to quit sugar, use natural, safe products, and eat fermented food is

178

tantamount to quackery? But putting tubes in the child's ear and keeping him permanently on antibiotics is normal?

The medical profession believes they have a monopoly on health the way the Catholic church tried to have a monopoly on God during the Dark Ages. You don't need to be Catholic (or any other religion for that matter) to talk to God, and you don't need your M.D. to get back to homeostatic health.

Getting back to the final domino of colon function: A common symptom of an unhealthy colon is constipation or loose bowels. If any domino is missing or is prevented from falling, it stops the entire chain throughout the digestive system. Constipation is literally a huge block to the digestive dominos falling. Where do you think food goes when it's not digested? When people say they are constipated for years, what do you think happens to all that compacted waste in the colon? Loose bowels and diarrhea are actually a form of constipation. When your bowels are completely backed up or toxic, the body will activate the diarrhea as a last-ditch effort to remove waste.

The natural, easy, and super effective answer to healthy bowel function is probiotic rich fermented foods. This, of course, after you have already eliminated sugar, processed foods, and carbohydrates from your diet.

PROBIOTICS & FERMENTED FOODS

It is imperative that you understand the importance of fermentation, microorganisms, and healthy bacteria. Even Louis Pasteur allegedly admitted "it is the microbes that will have the last word."

A healthy gut must be continuously reinforced with new bacteria (probiotics) and the food for the probiotics (prebiotics). A very concentrated tablet may have as many as 50 billion live bacteria. Yet one tablespoon of a fermented food can have as much as a trillion live bacteria and as many as 30 to 40 different strains.

Fermented foods are accorded near mystical powers in every human culture. They make you happy and extend your life. It is a documented, scientific fact that consuming oral probiotics will:[80]

- Reduce oxidative stress
- Decrease inflammatory markers
- Increase mental outlook on life
- Improve cognition

James Cook, Captain of a fleet for the British empire and the first person to circumnavigate the globe several times, sailed with barrels of sauerkraut for his crew to prevent scurvy and encourage strength.[81] In Hawaii, he ate case poi, a thick starchy fermented taro-root soup. According to stories, if the sailers would refuse the sauerkraut he would have them beaten, as he knew the importance of this superfood.

Abraham of the Bible consumed kefir and, I'm sure, it was one of the factors contributing to his long life and virility at old age. The word "kefir" is derived from the Turkish word "keif," which translates to the "good feeling" one has after drinking it. Ancient cultures have long known of the healing abilities of kefir. Kefir is a mildly sour and slightly carbonated fermented milk. The various types of beneficial bacteria contained in kefir make it one of the most potent probiotic foods available. Making your own is easy and it's like having a pet you care for!

Russian immunologist and Nobel laureate Eli Metchnikoff studied the eating habits of people who had reached the age of 100 in the Balkans and stated that Lactobacillus, "postpones and ameliorates old age."[82] Fermented foods clearly provide the necessary microbial diversity to make the digestive system resilient.

Yet modern day medicine continues its bacterial warfare unabated. Widespread antibiotic and antibacterial substance abuse only serves to kill the weakest bacteria and leads to the evolution of super germs. 80,000 people die in hospitals each year from infections acquired in the hospital by bacteria that are resistant to all known antibiotics.

The greatest threat to American health is the practice of destroying the gut and its microflora with antibiotics and antacids. Autoimmune diseases, strange viruses, antibiotic resistant bacteria, and allergies are the short list of diseases that result. The worst are the ugly, mutated antibiotic resistant offspring of this irresponsibility. Diseases like C-diff are ravaging hospitals and weakening patients. They are so bad that 10% of people that enter a hospital leave with an infection they didn't have when they entered[83].

Interestingly enough, the only treatment for this disease is a stool transplant. You take the stool from a healthy human, blend it up with saline water, and inject it into the suffering patient's colon. It's a proven remedy as a treatment for C-diff only, but studies are showing amazing results for a variety of other conditions like obesity, autoimmune disease, depression, allergies, etc.[84]

Think about it—if your bacterial gut biome controls your DNA function, it makes perfect sense to put a super concentrated source of healthy stool directly into the colon. I was so fascinated by this concept that I once begged my wife to whip up a batch in our blender so I could inject it into my colon, but she refused. If you're interested in this concept just go to YouTube and watch videos about people doing this. Like most amazing cures, it's easy and it's free.

The more sterile we live, the sicker we become. Too bad we've been told the opposite all our entire life, much to our collective health detriment. Sandor Ellix Katz in his book *Wild Fermentation* quotes Dr. David Rosenstreich, director of Allergy and Immunology at the Albert Einstein School of Medicine saying, "The cleaner we live...the more likely we'll get asthma and allergies."

Every healthy human culture ate fermented foods with almost every meal. It was known, without the scientific explanation, that these fermented foods made us stronger, prevented sickness, and improved well-being. Today we document scientifically that the incredible biodiversity of bacterial life and the ample enzymes contained in these foods are the reason for the positive mystical effect fermented foods.

Don't be fooled by the fake ferments. Most commercial yogurts and sauerkrauts are worthless. A yogurt that is fat-free and high in sugar is not healthy. It's disguised diabetes waiting to happen. If it tastes sweet, spit it out. Yogurt is sour. Most sauerkrauts have been "stabilized" to have no live bacteria. Heat kills bacteria. When you roast your ribs in store-bought kraut in a crock pot you kill bacteria. Make it yourself, eat it raw, and if you buy it in the store, make sure you buy the live, cultured kind.

Try to eat a fermented food each day and preferably with each meal. A little bit of the 5 K's - raw kraut, kombucha, kvass, kimchi, or kefir. These foods are delicious and powerful builders of health. If you don't like fermented food or don't have access to it, then use a good pre/probiotic supplement daily. Lastly, if there is an overgrowth of bad bacteria in the colon, remove it by a weed and feed protocol.

WEED AND FEED

If your gut is full of pathogenic bacteria, they must be eliminated before good bacteria can re-seed. The seats of your stadium need to be emptied of the foreign invading team before the home team fans can take the seats! The carbohydrate reset of no sugar will go a long way in doing this. Additionally, you will need to take an anti-pathogenic to clear the seats. Both my experience and studies show that oregano is the most potent and effective at accomplishing this.[85]

Here is how you will check if you need to take oregano: In the morning before eating anything, spit into a glass of water and perform the Candida Spit Test. (You may want to put out a glass of water on the bed stand or bathroom counter, just to remind yourself not to brush your teeth before spitting in the glass). Check the water every 15 minutes for up to one hour. Your saliva is carrying fungal overgrowth if you see strings (like legs) traveling down into the water from the saliva floating on the top or cloudy saliva that sinks to the bottom of the glass, or cloudy specks suspended in the water then the saliva is carrying a fungal overgrowth.

Did you see any of the above ___Yes ___No If yes: which: _____

183

Candida spit test

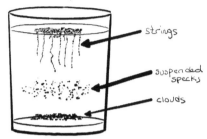

If your morning spit sinks as above, add in 100 mg oregano each morning and evening (50 mg for children) for the first week. After seven days, switch to probiotics. Be prepared. For many a reaction may occur as you kill off the bad bacteria and it's removed from the body. Many people will feel irritable, low energy, and sometimes even feverish. If the symptoms are more intense than you're willing to accept, lower the dose of oregano.

Summary of the Digestive Dominoes:
1. Stomach: look at symptoms and palplate, if positive perform stomach juice test—take 2 stomach juice tablets with each meal or apple cider vinegar every day with water.
2. Fill out liver symptoms, perform liver palpation test. If positive, take liver drainage tablets every day.
3. Perform a liver flush during the last week of the 21 days.
4. Take nine tablets of digestive enzymes every day. If you're very ill take 18.

5. Take six tablets of probiotics or eat fermented food every day

6. Do the spit test. If it's positive take oregano for the first week.

7. Try to get muscle tested for allergies and then use the Allergy Elimination Technique

Good. Now that we're grounded, let's get some air in us and move on to the next element!

oregano - 50 mg

17 - OXYGEN

ELEMENT—AIR

REMOVE: CO_2, mouth breathing and inactivity
ADD IN: Oxygen production plants in the home, diaphragm stretches, deep breathing, and aerobic exercise

OK, we got through the Earth Element. We've given up sugar, replaced our minerals, started eating organic and up-regulated our digestion. Now it's time we move on to the element of *air*, which is really the primary element we need for life. Just as fish swim in the sea, we swim in the air. Humans can go days without water and weeks without food, but just as a fish cannot live without water, we can only last a few short minutes with an improper air supply. Every cell in our body is in constant exchange with the outside, drinking oxygen and expelling acid, which we breath out via carbon dioxide. 70% of our metabolic acids left over from cellular metabolism are expelled through our breathing. Without proper understanding of the Air element, acids can accumulate and overwhelm the body.

Most people have never had the amazing feeling of having proper oxygen circulating through their bodies and full elimination of CO_2. After I teach people how to manage the Air element, many say that they feel so good they feel like they're high—high on life.

With increased man-made environmental changes, we have seen a decrease in the oxygen in our biosphere and an increase in air pollution. For most of known history, the oxygen level in our biosphere has been

186

around 35%[86], and within that last 100 years it has dropped to 20%.[87] In some cityscapes, smog hangs heavily and the oxygen can be as low as 11%. Forget about getting high, if you're breathing in polluted 11% oxygen air, you are going to feel terrible. The next few chapters will provide a succinct guide for understanding how to increase our Air for supercharging our bodies with living air and getting really high!

We will learn how to super oxygenate your body by:

- Creating clean, oxygenated air in your living space.
- Removing any restrictions in your diaphragm and lungs.
- Performing a breathing technique known as Oxygen Flush Breathing.
- Moving more and exercising correctly.

CLEAN, OXYGENATED AIR.

When breathing, it's of first importance to have clean, oxygenated air. Your lungs, unlike your bowels and skin, have no barrier to stop toxins from immediately entering your bloodstream. If you live in a metropolitan area like I do, pay special attention to this chapter and the breathing environment in which you live.

There is a huge problem today with air pollution inside houses and office buildings. The chemically treated lumber, flooring, carpeting, paint, and adhesives release enormous amounts of carcinogenic gaseous molecules that pile onto our allostatic stress load. To add to this problem, newly designed energy efficient buildings actually trap indoor pollutants and CO_2, making the problem worse.

City air quality is deplorable. Smokestacks spew forth toxic burn-off, and cars cough smoke from their exhaust while there is little to no plant life to counteract and clean the air. As a result, most homes and office spaces in industrialized areas have very low oxygen levels. This problem is only made worse when there are multiple people occupying a living space and/or it's wintertime.

The first and most obvious step in healing our Air element is to increase oxygen within our living space. Since oxygen is the natural byproduct of plant photosynthesis, it stands to reason that we should have more plants in our home or live closer to nature. By filling our living space with oxygen producing plants that clean the air, we can improve our blood oxygen levels and reduce our exposure to toxins. NASA has done extensive research on this topic, and found that the addition of common household plants can trap toxins, eliminate excessive carbon dioxide, and increase oxygen levels.

The NASA Clean Air study found that certain plants can trap almost all outgassing from toxins, such as carpets, paint, and synthetic compounds, while other plants can produce high amounts of oxygen. In this research they found that 15-18 high oxygen producing plants in 6-8 inch pots will sufficiently improve air quality in an 1,800 square foot home. This means that for every 100 square feet of living space we should have a large planted pot. It was found certain household plants are so efficient at cleaning and oxygenating the air that if your house was placed in an air-tight bubble with no input of oxygen or release of CO_2, these plants would provide enough oxygen for you to breathe completely while simultaneously eliminating all the CO_2. Amazing.[88]

You may not feel you need as many plants in your home as NASA found necessary, but it's still important to incorporate as many as possible. You'll soon find indoor plants make a living space more...livable. Or, you'll also find that moving closer to nature and planting more trees around your home makes your life more beautiful. The following is a short list of plants that have been shown to be especially beneficial in the home. Feel free to decorate with whatever works in your environment and that you find beautiful, since all plants produce oxygen.

BEST PLANTS FOR A HOME

1. Areca Palm (Chrysalidocarpus Lutescens)

This plant is efficient at converting CO_2 back into oxygen and cleaning pollutants from the air. This plant grows well in filtered light and needs to be watered often.

2. Snake Plant (Sansevieria trifasciata)

This plant is often called "The Bedroom Plant" as it produces oxygen at night. This plant does well in full or filtered light and doesn't need to be watered often.

3. Money Plant (Epipremnum aureum)

This plant has been shown by NASA to remove chemicals and other pollutants from the home. It does well in filtered light with light watering. This plant is toxic to animals and children so be careful and try to place this plant high up where the little ones can't get to it.

After you are in an oxygenated living space, now you have to breathe that oxygen in!

GET THE OXYGEN IN THE BODY

I remember one day back when I was sick when I was standing in my bathroom looking in the mirror. I had just coughed up a glob of mucus, which I did almost every night as I had been fighting a chronic cough for years.

And then it happened. I had a breakthrough and a major turning point in my life. While standing there I decided to take a deep breath in, stand up straight and push my chest out. As I did I felt a sharp pull through my chest, from my right lung down to my liver. Wanting to fight through this I stood up even straighter, but as I did I got extremely lightheaded, passed out and fell onto the bathroom floor. When I came to I thought about what had just happened and immediately realized that I had a restriction in my lungs and diaphragm, limiting me from breathing deeply. This started me on a journey of discovery.

Thinking I might have lung cancer I immediately took an x-ray of my lungs which, thankfully, were clear. After ruling out cancer, I started researching every breathing, diaphragm, and lung stretch that I could find. Surprisingly, I found that there is a lack of information how to free up the diaphragm and lungs. There are hundreds of thousands of pages dedicated to Pokémon, but very few on how to breathe. Over the years, since that moment in the bathroom, I have been working on putting together my own protocol for the Air element. I am proud to say that I found the solution and made a major discovery in healing.

Following my own protocol has changed my life. Moving and breathing in the ways I'll describe in this chapter, will allow light and oxygen to infuse and fill you. As you open up your chest and lungs, a new way of being will emerge in you. The information in this chapter will change your life if you apply it.

The following techniques are based in-part on chiropractic principles, yoga techniques, a breathing technique called the Wim Hoff method, and a technique called Holotrophic breathing. I have combined and incorporated theses sources in a way that works incredibly well at oxygenating the body to the deepest level. Please don't skip this step, as it's a part of the formula.

Alright, let's get more oxygen into our bodies and learn to breath fully and without restriction. Since that day in the bathroom and the discovery of a method of releasing the chest and lungs, I have started examining the diaphragms of all my patients. I have found that most people with health issues have a frozen diaphragm, which makes them unable to fully and effectively breathe deeply. Like a black hole, a frozen diaphragm pulls everything into it. First the shoulders are pulled forward, then the head, and finally it brings our entire upper body into a state of flexion. Imagine right now what an old sick person looks like when they stand or walk. Are they upright, shoulders back, chest open, looking forward? No! They are flexed forward, their head is down, and they look at the ground when they walk. A chronic spasm of the diaphragm always accompanies sickness and aging. Doing the techniques in this chapter will help you fight against it and will slow the aging process.

The diaphragm is one of the largest muscles in the body. When it contracts, it pulls the lungs down, which expands them and sucks air into the body. When we don't take full breaths with our diaphragm, we are progressively reducing oxygen in the body and increasing acid waste. This acid slowly fills our muscles, organs and plasma and creates cascading detrimental side effects

191

including changes in mood, brain fog, increased pain, and increased fat deposits, always ending in disease. Even if it's only a 5% reduction in breath, it will lead to a 5% reduction in our cells' ability to function. On the flip side, a 5% increase in function can add years of good living to one's life.

Most people have far more than a 5% reduction and I estimate that low energy, sick people have at least a 50% reduction in diaphragm movement and strength. People with extremely low energy, chronic disease and cancer often have a completely frozen diaphragm. This is clearly evident from their posture, their acidic pH, and short breath holding time that most have on examination.

Factors that contribute to poor diaphragm movement and spasm and therefore oxygen starvation throughout the body are:

- Chronic cough
- Smoking
- Chronic vomiting
- Sitting too much
- Emotional burdens—we tend to quit breathing when emotionally traumatized and then these traumas are stored within our diaphragm
- Pregnancy pushing up on the diaphragm
- A difficult birth resulting in an improper first breath of life
- Simply never being shown how to breathe properly.

There are four simple tests you can do to determine the state of your breathing function. Test your breath holding time right now and see how long you can hold your breath. Then measure the pH of your saliva and see how much accumulated metabolic acids you have built up. Look at your posture and finally move your stomach up and down and see how free your diaphragm is.

How long can your breath? _____

When one is properly consuming and adsorbing nutrition (food, water, air) and expelling metabolic waste, an individual should be able to hold their breath for at least one minute, but ideally at least two minutes. The time that you can hold your breath is one of the best predictors of overall health. The more built up metabolic acids you have and restriction in your chest, the less oxygenated you are and the shorter your breath holding time will be. Anything less that 30 seconds is a sign of severe acidosis of the body.

What is the pH of your saliva? _____

As stated in the mineral chapter, as you become progressively more acidic due to low minerals and high acids, the pH of the salvia will turn acidic. There is not any one thing that corrects pH. You must quit sugar, consume more minerals and learn to breathe properly. Since most of the acid is removed via your lungs, the breath work in this chapter is a must. The pH of the saliva should ideally be 7.2.

How does your posture look? Test your posture against a wall, how many inches forward is your head? _____

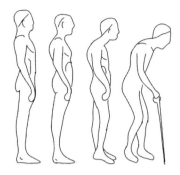

Stand comfortably with a wall at your back right now, then have someone measure how far you head is forward from the wall. If your posture is correct with an open chest and diaphragm your calves, butt, shoulder blades and the back of your head should all touch the wall at the same time. If they are not, you need to work on opening your chest and diaphragm.

Move your diaphragm up and down and see how free the movement is.

Lie on your back on the floor and place a book on your tummy. Breathe in and out deeply and try to make the book rise with your breath in and drop with your breath out. The book should move at least four inches up and down, how much is your's moving? _____

THE SOLUTIONS TO RESTRICTED BREATH

Let's first start with the basics. Breathing should begin with nose and flow to the belly, not from the mouth to the chest. Mouth breathers have been shown to have an entire host of negative physical effects, including slowed mental function[89]. A proper breath should come in through the nose, the diaphragm should drop, and as it expands down the belly should come out.

Ever notice how a healthy baby breathes? Slowly, deeply, with it's belly. Use that image when focusing on your breathing. Breathe slowly and deeply, breathe through your nose to your diaphragm. Do not lift your shoulders and chest with your breath. Keep your shoulders and chest relaxed. Bring your belly in and slowly exhale. Why? When you extend your belly, you are creating space to expand your lungs into the abdomen, opening up your lungs and capturing additional oxygen. When your belly comes in on expiration, it assists the lungs in expelling CO_2 and other gaseous waste. Make all effort to avoid being a mouth breather.

The fascia, which is the soft tissue network that holds together the entire body, is deeply attached to the diaphragm. The constant, slow dropping of the diaphragm assists the unwinding of the fascial twists in the body. By fixing your breath, you're also fixing your diaphragm. By fixing your diaphragm, you oxygenate your cells. By oxygenating your cells, you increase function. By increasing their function, you improve your cellular environment and therefore your level of health. These enhancements can all be accomplished in two simple steps on the way to mastery.

STEP 1 - DIAPHRAGM STRETCHES

To fix a spasmed diaphragm, perform the following three stretches. Do each stretch 10 minutes per day, then do the Oxygen Flush Breathing described below. These should be done in the morning as soon as you wake up.

STRETCH #1
While lying on your back, flat on the ground (with no pillow), place an object on your belly and breathe as deeply as you are able, making the object go up when you breathe in and down when you breathe out. As you practice this technique, you will be able to lift the object higher and higher with each breath in. When I first began doing this breathing I was barely able to lift my abdomen at all, and over a period of weeks I became able to move the object over four inches. As I was doing this I felt as though I was ripping up adhesions in my chest and stomach. It's OK to work through pain—you won't do any damage with deep breathing. Spend 10 minutes focusing on your breath and expanding your belly with your breath as much as you're able. Then move on to warm up exercise #2.

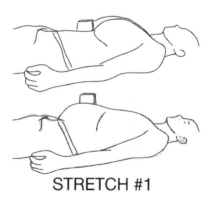

STRETCH #1

STRETCH #2

Then sit up, knees crossed, and take several large of breaths in and out before taking in as large of a breath as you can and holding it in. Once the breath is fully in and you can't take in any more air, sit up as straight as you're able and push your belly out as much as you can, expand your chest, and look up at the sky. Hold your breath and this position for 10-20 seconds and stretch open your chest and diaphragm. WARNING: As this is a powerful way of opening up adhesions in the lungs and diaphragm, you will most likely get lightheaded when you first begin doing this. This is because you are hyper-oxygenating the body. My personal experience when I first began this was that I would get so lightheaded that I often would fall over. I got the idea of how to do this from passing out in the bathroom years earlier. This is why I highly recommend doing this while sitting. Expect to get lightheaded. Embrace it, knowing that you are opening your lungs and ripping through old adhesions. Perform 10-20 repetitions of this.

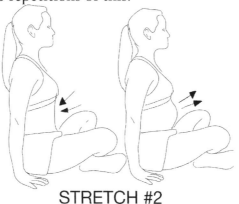

STRETCH #2

STRETCH #3

Finally, what I call the golden movement. It is the motion of rising up and opening yourself. When done properly, it's the most powerful motion I've ever encountered. You won't understand what I mean until you try this.

I discovered the golden movement one day in yoga class while trying to move and hold my breath in a way to expand my lungs. While I was in the downward dog yoga position, I took several large breaths in and out, then took in as much air as I was able and held the breath in as I moved into the upward dog yoga position. I wasn't prepared for what happened next. As soon as I got into the upward dog position, while still holding my breath and stretching open my chest, I felt like I got hit with a tornado of energy.

I saw geometric shapes, I felt my parasympathetic nervous system exploding with energy, and a wave of insights hit...then I passed out...again. I was only out for maybe 5 seconds but when I came to I realized I had found the answer I was seeking.

Over the next three months I repeated the entire breathing protocol described here and did the golden movement each day. During that time I dropped 20 pounds of inflammation off my body, all the pain and old injuries almost magically disappeared, joy came back into my life, and my brain function exploded.

I realize now that I had deep adhesion through my right lung, my diaphragm, and my liver. With these exercises I was able to open them up and begin to breathe again. It was only after opening my chest that I understood that my chest and breathing had been frozen ever since I experienced the car accident as a child.

Many of us store old injuries in our diaphragm. When we get hurt physically or emotionally, we tend to hold our breath and contract the diaphragm. Over time it quits moving completely. As it does, we begin to recruit our upper chest muscles to do the breathing, only sucking in a fraction of the oxygen we should be getting.

To get in this stretch, get in the downward dog position (pictures below) and take in 10 deep breaths. On the 10th breath, suck in as much air as you're able and hold your breath in. Then, move into the upward facing dog position. Try to expand and open your chest and belly as much as you can, then look up to the sky. When you first start, you will probably get lightheaded. Try to work through this feeling, fight to hold the position, fight to open your chest and lungs as much as you can, and hold the upward dog position and your breath for at least 20 seconds. The feeling will bring on intense imagery while it awakens your nervous and vascular systems.

This is powerful and intense healing. When beginning this you will get an oxygen flush, see stars, and have an immediate change in your state. As you remove the restrictions in your lungs, the experiences will get less intense. Try to work up to five repetitions.

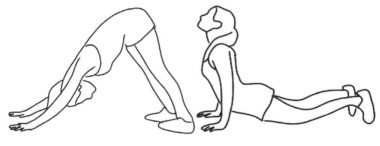

STRETCH #3

STEP 2 - OXYGEN FLUSH BREATHING
(OFB)

Once you have mastered focusing on your breath and opening up your chest, lungs, and diaphragm, you can then begin to oxygenate the body to fire up your cellular function. You know how when you blow on coals in a campfire they glow, get hotter, and burn brighter? Our cells respond in the same way to oxygen flush breathing.

Our cells' engines need to have oxygen, just like a burning ember, and our bodies do everything they can to saturate with as much oxygen as possible for optimal function. As we become oxygenated, first our red blood cells become saturated, then the oxygen fills up the intracellular plasma, and finally our tissues.

When we're under stress, our bodies divert oxygen to only the most important functions, like our extremities so we can fight or flee. First, oxygen and blood flow are pulled away from our spleen and immune system, then our digestive tract and liver, and finally away from our vascular system and brain.

As extensively covered in the first half of this book, our bodies need to *recover* from this stress response for us to return to homeostasis. It does this by activating the **para**sympathetic system. Think of it like a **para**chute slowing us down. The parasympathetic system is designed to help us recover after the stressful event and divert blood back to our vital organs. The problem is that, for our parasympathetic system to work properly, the stress (physical, emotional, chemical burdens) needs to go away and we need to have lots of oxygen, fat, and minerals for it to draw upon. For most of us that day never comes.

As a result, we get stagnation in the blood cells. They become stiff, blocking small capillaries throughout the body. With this blockage, areas of tissue become starved for oxygen and go into a type of hibernation. In this state of oxygen hibernation they can only burn sugar and produce acid. This is how inflammation and disease works.

With OFB you will activate your parasympathetic system, begin to break through old areas of blood stagnation throughout the body and return blood flow and oxygen to regions of your body that have been shut down for years. As this occurs, you will shed years of weight and inflammation from your body.

As you do this, you will first find that your digestion will start to improve as blood flow and oxygen return to your liver and bowels. You will then notice your immune system begin to improve as your vascular system and spleen function turns back on and recycles old stagnant blood. Finally, you'll feel your brain function, mood, and level of joy begin to increase.

Breathing deeply and performing OFB will change your life. I don't say it lightly. OFB is the next step to taking your health to a higher level. Perform OFB after doing the three diaphragm stretches each day. OFB, simply explained, is you breathe deeply and heavily for an extended period of time with periods of breath holding. This process first works to increase the oxygen in your blood and plasma through rapid breathing and then as you hold your breath, the blood vessels and capillaries slam open in an effort to get rid of CO_2. As they do this, you breathe deeply again and oxygenate deeper into your body. Repeat this process over and over until your body is fully oxygenated. Do this every day during your 21-day reset.

OXYGEN FLUSH BREATHING INSTRUCTIONS:

- On the first round, breathe in and out through your nose for 60 repetitions. For the first 20, breathe at a normal pace. For the second 20, hyperventilate as quickly as you are able. For the last 20, breathe as slowly and deeply as you are able.
- After the 60th breathe, take a huge breath in and hold it as long as you are able.
- After you can't hold it any longer, breathe out and recover.
- As soon as you recover, take another 60 repetitions through and out the nose.
- Then breathe out and hold your breath out. When you feel like you can't hold it another second, try to hold it another 10 seconds and then another 10! Hold it until you feel like you're going to pass out.
- Then, take as large a breath in as you can and hold it as long as possible.
- Let it out when you can't hold it any longer. Take a couple of breaths to recover and then repeat the entire process.
- On the second round, repeat the same process, but breathe in through your nose and out through your mouth.
- On the third round, repeat the same process, but breathe in through your mouth and out through your mouth.

It is important to time how long your can hold your breath. With each round you should be able to hold your breath longer. As you heal your diaphragm, oxygenate your body, and remove built up acids, you will be able to work up to holding your breath for 2-3 minutes. When I first started these exercises I couldn't hold my breath more than 45 seconds. Now on the third round I can frequently hold my breath for three minutes.

What I find interesting is that my breath-holding time will vary greatly based on what I ate the previous day. If I eat junk food and drink beer, which I rarely do, my breath-holding time drops by half. This simple observation is a testament to how toxic- and acid-forming these carbohydrates are to the body.

Additionally, many have speculated that this type of breathing naturally releases DMT (dimethyltryptamine) in your pineal gland. This is often associated with deep meditative states, opening of the "third eye" and spiritual breakthroughs. After the third round it becomes very easy to go into a deep meditative state for a period of time. During this time, simply become aware of what you feel, shut off your thoughts, focus on your breath and allow your body to go into a healing state.

The healing from this breath work is remarkable and intense. I've worked with grown men who have broken down in tears as they experience deep healing and life realizations. Some people visualize going back into their lives and working through traumas. People often report the sensation of going through the birthing process.

The diaphragm stretches and OFB breathing will take approximately 45-60 minutes. We frequently like to make excuses for why we don't have time to work on our bodies, but doing this you will literally add time to your day and life. As your brain and nervous system come into balance you will find yourself easily working through your to-do lists and accomplishing tasks that formerly seemed impossible. You will quickly become aware of increased energy, mental focus, feeling more centered, positivity and a host of other improvements. This 60 minutes will be the best 60 minutes of your day.

18 - MOVEMENT

ELEMENT—AIR

REMOVE: A sedentary lifestyle
ADD IN: 10,000 aerobic movements per day

After you breathe, you must move. Life is movement, and only upon death does movement stop. I don't need to tell you this. Time and again, studies prove that healthy people move and unhealthy people don't. According to a CBS News report, the CDC states that 80% of Americans don't get enough exercise.[90] Translation: 80% of Americans do not move on a daily basis in any meaningful manner, and therefore 80% of Americans are unhealthy. How un-American! Movement is so critical to health because it is responsible for circulating lymph and removing waste fluids.

Many of us wake up in our comfortable beds and take about 10 steps to get in our car and drive to work before continuing to sit at our desks until lunch. At lunch we go to the break room or a restaurant where we sit while someone else prepares our lunch. We come back to work and sit at our desks until it is time to sit in our car for another round of rush hour, so we can sit and watch TV until we pass out. Next day it's wash, rinse, repeat. We sure do sit a lot.

An April 17, 2011 article in the *New York Times* titled "Is sitting a lethal activity?" said, "**Sitting is the new smoking.**"[91] The article examined the collaborated research of Doctors Levine and M. Jensen from the Mayo Clinic. The intent of the controlled six-year study was to find a reason for different metabolic rates amongst people. What they stumbled upon was that the group that didn't gain weight actually moved more. Dr. Jensen said, "The people who didn't gain weight were unconsciously moving around more. They hadn't started exercising more—that was prohibited by the study. Their bodies simply responded naturally by making more little movements...like taking the stairs, trotting down the hall to the office water cooler, bustling about with chores at home or simply fidgeting. On average, the subjects who gained weight sat two hours more per day than those who hadn't."

Lack of movement, also known as a sedentary lifestyle, is a disease of modern commerce. Nowadays, we flip out our iPhone and Chinese food is delivered to the door 30 minutes later. No preparation required. No need to walk to the barn and milk the cow, then go dig up a potato, and hunt down a wild hog. Today, it's the drive-through window.

Movement, or the lack thereof, changes gene expression. I've met twins where one is rock-solid and muscular and the other is a flabby mess. How is this possible when they have the same genetics? Take that rock-solid man and put him in bed for 30 days because of an illness or surgery, and he will "lose" all of his fitness and muscle tone.

The New England Journal of Medicine published an article in 2000 reporting on what investigators from the Karolinska Institute in Sweden found on a study of 44,788 pairs of twins. The study showed identical twins do not experience cancer at the same rate. They stated, "**Inherited genetic factors make a minor contribution to susceptibility to most types of neoplasms**," indicating that the environment has the principal role in causing cancer.[92]

Are you beginning to get the greater thread that runs throughout this book? Terrain is everything! Our lives are not the result of genetics beyond our control, but rather genetic expression of our lifestyle and within our ability to modify and change.

Over the last 50 years, volumes have been written on how we should move, lift, run, and dance ourselves into a state of fitness. In a matter of months, some people argue that we can have the body of our dreams if we just commit to an hour and a half of high-intensity resistance training every day. Some say we can cross-fit ourselves into supermen and women, while others still say we should just dance or jazzer-size ourselves to fitness. The funny thing is they're all right, with some strong caveats.

Instead of adding to all this "fitness" information, I choose to simplify it. Depending on your health, and how far you want to go with it, you need to progress through 2 easy steps with your fitness.

1. MOVE MORE
2. EXERCISE AEROBICALLY

1. MOVE MORE

When I was nine years old, my parents dropped me off at scout camp. We hiked every single day. In the morning, we would don 30 pound backpacks, clipping them onto our waists and shoulders. Ten miles later, we unpacked our junk, set up camp, and crashed. Upon waking up in the same spot where we collapsed into sleep, we packed up and hiked another 10 miles. We repeated this for 10 days. I, as you may perceive by my tone, despised it. It was miserable. I felt like I was being punished for a crime. My parents, on the other hand, thought it would be great exercise for their rambunctious young boy. I hated it, but they were right.

Today I love to hike because it's my choice and not a forced army march.

The first key is simple: move more. The key to sustained movement is joy. So find a movement that you truly enjoy. If you love to dance, dance every night. If you love to swim or surf, do it every day. My 70-year-old mother loves to garden, so she created a garden 10 times bigger than she needs and gives away the food. Just move and work to fall in love with your movement. The most essential yet basic of all movements is walking. Walking, from an evolutionary standpoint, is useful in our search for food, water, safe housing, and sex. Well, maybe some us run for sex. Walking enlivens our social life as we go for a romantic walk or visit a neighbor/friend. Without walking, other human functions such as speaking, hearing, and touch eventually diminish.

This walking movement is required for a myriad of necessary functions. It infuses our lungs with life-giving oxygen. Arteries transport oxygen-rich red blood cells from our lungs to our tissues. Oxygen infusion improves circulation, decreases tissue aging, and literally makes our body "hard" and resistant to disease by stimulating our cells to grow in strength.

With movement, oxygen is exchanged for cellular waste and carbon dioxide, which we'll call cell poop. That poop is dumped into our lymphatic water system which then is eventually disposed of through various methods. Movement of our limbs and torso powers the efficiency of the lymphatic pumping system. The impact on our joints and muscles stresses cellular mechanoreceptors, resulting in strong and dense bones. Movement aids the brain's neuroplasticity, improving brain function, immune function, and digestion.

Movement is the basis of our evolution and none of the other elements in the body can function without sufficient movement. When humans ventured into space for prolonged periods, scientists quickly noticed rapid decay of the musculoskeletal system in their astronauts. Muscles shrank. Bone density disappeared at an alarming rate. They basically devolved. This is the biggest challenge for space exploration. Astronauts returning from the moon were barely able to walk on Earth and convalesced for elongated periods. As it turns out, gravity and our resistance to it is in essence the definition of movement and is absolutely imperative to our total well-being.

As a society, however, we strive to move less and less. Modern comforts make us obscenely docile. Here is your first challenge when it comes to movement: **Find a way to incorporate more movement into your life.** Remember that we need to move more than modern day life requires so you are going to have to find activities to add. My father's knees gave out over 20 years ago, yet he has found joy in adventuring and kayaking beautiful streams and lakes. He's in great shape at 70 years of age, and as far as I know has not been in a gym for years. What makes my soul sing is hiking through a lush forest. I love the oxygen-rich greenery moving past me. It really doesn't matter what you do, just do something. Take your bike to work, park farther away at the store, get a dog and go for a walk every night, buy a standing treadmill desk—just find ways to move more!

I love personal movement trackers as a way of holding us accountable on our movement. A minimum goal should be 10,000 movements per day and 70,000 per week. My wife averages around 20,000 movements per day working with horses and she is the most beautiful and fit person I have ever met.

I find the only way to get sufficient movement is with a movement tracker. Buy one of these right now and, during the first 21 days, make sure that you are doing at least 10,000 movements per day. No excuses.

Remember, do whatever you enjoy but make sure you get in 10,000 movements! Do this for a couple of weeks and when you're ready to up your game and exercise, then you can move on to step #2.

2. EXERCISE PROPERLY

Alright, are you ready to exercise? This is where the education has to begin because many of the current approaches to exercise that have been co-opted by self-proclaimed gurus, TV shows, and salesmen are mostly wrong. Some of them genuinely think they know the answer and sell us gimmicky diets or hardware. Others try to educate through entertainment and create ridiculous extreme makeover shows like "The Biggest Loser." The approach in these shows is to shove some poor obese guy on a treadmill and scream at him for "motivation." Sometimes the weight comes off. Most times, the weight comes back. These gurus pretend weight gain is nothing more than overeating and laziness. "Calories in, calories out," they ignorantly shout.

As a response, we flock to gyms to lift weights and run in place. The typical gym promotes platitudes like the "no pain, no gain" method of exercise. I'm always mystified by this "pain" philosophy. I watch bemusedly as people push themselves to agonized exhaustion, often with someone hanging over them encouraging more pain. Wall graffiti in the gym might proclaim something like "pain is weakness leaving the body" or "only the strong survive." Men grunt, flex, and stare at themselves in the mirror, while women hang on to the treadmill for dear life. Magazines are scattered throughout the gym. The covers display airbrushed pictures of unattainable bodies. Motivated to achieve this impossible standard, most push right up to the breaking point. As people sense the impending breakage, they use caffeine, nitro, sugar, or some other stimulant like anabolic steroids to get through their workouts. If you need these, your adrenal stress glands are already exhausted. Exhaustion and substance-abuse leads to a collapse, generally followed by a prolonged illness. It's guaranteed to happen. It's clearly documented scientific fact that they are exchanging fitness for health.

Some of us exercise to push the boundaries of our bodies in an attempt to feel fully alive as the adrenaline pumps through us. Something like being face-to-face with a grizzly bear. The adrenaline turns on and our senses heighten, we feel each bead of sweat roll down our brow and pause on our nose tip before falling in slow motion to the ground. We notice the sweet-scented mountain breeze ruffle every hair of the bear, we hear our breath, we hear the bear growl, we feel our heart beat. Time seems to practically halt as we watch the bear's eyes. Though we are scared, we are awed and we are alive. We then either run like hell or fight the bear to the death.

In an attempt to re-create adrenaline rushes like this, many of us like to push exercise to the very brink of exhaustion every time. We run a marathon, do the spartan races, and try to join the Crossfit games. We push as hard as we can, thinking, believing, and hoping like hell this is going to bring us health. I too believed this was the answer and once did the Chicago Marathon. It was the most painful experience of my life. The finish line looked like a medical nightmare. People sprawled out half-dead everywhere, the medical tent full of people gasping on oxygen machines with IVs hanging in their arms. I was on crutches for a week. Many of these athletes, though being fit, are not healthy.

From a scientific point of view, when we push to exhaustion it excites the adrenals, pulling sugar reserves for fuel to burst forth into an explosion of energy. When they get worn out from too much exercise or anaerobic stress, energy production quickly diminishes. Fatigue is the first sign of this syndrome. It's our body's gentle way of saying, "Please, let me rest." Disrespecting the body's message, we tell our adrenals to suck it up and we keep pushing our body to the limits with a smattering of addictive substances. These substances whip the tired horse, and for a while it works. For a while.

Our body is only capable of a limited amount of adrenaline responses before we break. Then we wanna-be athletes wonder why our knees and back give out when we're 30, or we suffer from chronic fatigue by the time we hit 35. Racked with injuries and pain, we quit exercise completely.

Before any exercise regime can begin, it is imperative that adrenal health is tested and restored. Do not exercise intensely if you are in Phase III of adrenal stress exhaustion. You need rest in this state. Go for a walk.

Once your adrenals are working and you're ready to start exercising, I'll describe how you can do it so you maximize cellular function. You can turn your cellular engines into red hot coals pumping out constant energy. I'm going to teach you how to exercise so that you don't get injured, and I'm going to show you how to exercise so there is very little pain but the results are the best you've ever gotten. But before I do all this, let's first ensure your adrenals are ready for it with a simple home test called Ragland's blood pressure test. Exercising before your adrenals are ready will only lead to more dysfunction. Perform the following test right now:

RAGLAND'S BLOOD PRESSURE TEST

The regulation of the blood pressure is an easy way to measure both cardiac and adrenal function. For those unfamiliar, the adrenals are two walnut-sized glands that sit on top of each of your kidneys. They are central to our exercise and stress response system and perform necessary functions such as blood sugar regulation, blood pressure regulation and production of cortisol and adrenaline. It's essential these little puppies are working properly before you add the additional stress of exercise.

Since one of the adrenals' functions is blood pressure regulation with moving, this allows us to easily and accurately test them. If your adrenals are working properly, then your blood pressure should go up a little bit when you go from laying to standing. If it drops, it's a sign the adrenal glands are exhausted and are unable to perform their duty. Performing this test on yourself can help you know when you need to rest, take a break from exercise, and start supplementation. (By the way, you can do this without a blood pressure cuff too. Just lay down on the ground for a couple of minutes and then stand up quickly. Did you get really light headed for a few seconds? If you did, your adrenal glands are exhausted and you're not ready to push the machine too hard yet. Go for a walk instead.)

The Ragland's blood pressure test measures adrenal fatigue as a function of blood pressure. It's simple to do on your own. There are two easy steps for the Ragland's blood pressure test.

1. Take your blood pressure lying down.
2. Stand up quickly and take your blood pressure again immediately.

HOW TO READ THE RESULTS:

Blood pressure is given with two different numbers. The top number is your *systolic pressure* and indicates the highest pressure of blood movement through your body. The bottom number is your *diastolic pressure* and indicates the residual pressure between contractions of the heart. This difference between the two is your *pulse pressure*. So for example if your blood pressure is 130/90 (mm Hg) then your pulse pressure is 40. Anything greater than 40 is abnormal and can potentially indicate heart fatigue created by nutritional deficiencies (primarily B, C vitamins and CoEnzyme Q10). A pulse pressure of over 60 indicates a high risk of cardiovascular disease, heart attack, or congestive heart failure. If your pulse pressure is over 60, your systolic is over 160, or you diastolic is over 100, you should definitely *not* try to exercise. Instead go for a walk and begin supplementation immediately. I recommend a product called Heart Food by Whole Body Health or one called Cardio Plus by Standard Process.

If your blood pressure stays the same or rises when you stand then you have healthy adrenals and the vital function of getting blood and oxygen to your brain is working properly. If your blood pressure drops as you stand up, your adrenals are fatigued. You must rest and take a break from exercise. If you don't rest, your risk of injury and breakdown is greatly enhanced. Go for a walk.

If your blood pressure dropped and you got lightheaded when you stood up, then you must add an adrenal support supplement to your supplement regime until you have recovered your energy and your Ragland's blood pressure test. For adrenal support, I use a product called Adrenal Food by Whole Body Health with great success. Another great one is by a company called Standard Process called Drenemin.

213

These free tests are highly effective measurements and every doctor and health warrior should perform them.

What's your:

Reclining Blood Pressure _____.

Standing Blood Pressure _____

Pulse Pressure_____

Do you need to add in an additional adrenal or heart supplements?

Yes _____ No _____ Which? _____

Once these are normal, then begin aerobic exercise:

AEROBIC EXERCISE

Sweetness! You're already moving 10,000 steps per day, your adrenal function is restored and you're ready to up your game. Let's do this...but properly. As a physician, I think only about what improves overall cellular function and health. Regardless of how we choose to exercises, it's important when exercising to do it in a way that doesn't destroy our hormonal system or inhibit our cellular ability to take up nutrition and oxygen in exchange for energy.

As stated in the carbohydrate reset chapter, burning fat is 80 times more efficient than burning sugar. Fat efficiently powers all movement. The fat we store during days of abundance serves as fuel. Most of us have enough fat reserves to run hundreds of miles without stopping, though we may lack the muscle strength and endurance to do it.

For our cells to burn this fat, the Krebs cycle requires sufficient oxygen to be present. This is known as aerobic metabolism. Sometimes, however, the aerobic (with oxygen) fat burning Krebs cycle in our cells cannot keep up with the requirements of oxygen needed during periods of extreme output. Our infinitely wise bodies solve this by converting our fuel burning system to an anaerobic (without oxygen) process that burns sugar. This change allows for short bursts of extreme energy. In this anaerobic process, the adrenals issue cortisol to enable sugar to be released. Glycogen (sugar in the liver) is burned up first, followed by sugar from within the cells. Sugar produces lactic acid in exchange for extreme output.

As we perform anaerobic exercise, blood is diverted away from our vital organs. This high output process is known as the flight or fight mechanism and, evolutionary speaking, it enabled our ancestors to hunt and flee effectively.

The cells in our body develop based on what type of activity we perform on a regular basis. *This is important, so listen up*! If we exercise primarily anaerobically, we develop Type II cells that are designed to burn sugar. If we exercise primarily aerobically, we develop Type I cells that are designed to burn fat. Sort of like how a turkey has two colored muscles, we have two types of muscle fibers. These fibers are mixed in all of our muscles depending on how we move. Can you guess what type of cells I want you to develop so that you can become a fat burning machine?

The term aerobic was coined by a Dr. Kenneth Cooper in a book he wrote in 1968 called *Aerobics*. Dr. Cooper had been working with astronauts and was looking for the best form of movement to protect the government's investment. What he stumbled upon was groundbreaking. Just as avoiding sugar turns on your fat-burning hormone glucagon, aerobic exercise within a specific heart rate range massively oxygenates the body and builds up the efficiency of fat burning cells. As you exercise in this way, your mitochondrial function will improve and you'll have more energy.

This concept was proven and can be easily tested with a gas analyzer by measuring how much oxygen you consume versus carbon dioxide you expire. The more CO_2 you expire, the more you are burning sugar and producing acids. This increased acid invariably leads to inflammation and adrenal burn out. Inevitably, unhealthy, and diseased people burn more sugar for energy than fat. You can do this without a gas analyzer by simple performing the MAF test listed later to gauge how well your mitochondria generates energy.

Since we're trying to get the acid out and turn you into a low-inflammation, fat-burning machine, we must focus on building type I aerobic cells as much as humanly possible. Make sense? Also, as a bonus, since aerobics is not stressful to your adrenal glands, the incidence of injury drops dramatically.

The simplest way to know when you are building up the correct type of muscles is through the use of a heart rate monitor. A heart rate monitor effectively monitors between anaerobic or aerobic exercise by accurately keeping track of your heart rate. When you go above a certain heart rate, your oxygen cannot keep up and your body begins to convert over to sugar burning muscles. It's that simple.

A lot of people mistakenly think that aerobic exercise is running while weight lifting is anaerobic. This is a misconception, since oxygen content is all that matters. The type of exercise doesn't matter. Run, lift weights, bike, golf, make love. Go ahead! Perform any type of exercise you like, but stay right at or below your max aerobic heart rate.

Warning: When you first begin aerobically with a heart rate monitor, it's going to feel like you are exercising insanely slow and the cheetah in you is going to be restless. Just trust the process and I promise within a couple of months you will be moving quickly again, but at a much lower heart rate.

If you're doing an activity that requires that you go above your max aerobic heart rate, such as a heavy weightlifting set, simply let your body recover back to aerobic before you perform the next set. A reasonable goal for quantity of aerobic exercise is two hours per week.

It's that easy to maximize your fat burning! Saturate your body with oxygen!

DETERMINING YOUR MAX HEART RATE

A heart rate monitor and movement tracker are essential tools for any seasoned or would-be athlete and can both found in a single watch. Both Fitbit and Garmin make devices available for less than $150. This is money well spent. A heart rate monitor is the best trainer ever and is always with you.

There are lots of formulas out there to determine maximum aerobic heart rate, but the one described by Dr. Phil Maffatone in his book *In fitness and in Health* makes the most sense. His formula is as follows: Take 180 and subtract your age = maximum aerobic heart rate. So, if you're 46, subtract it from 180. Your maximum heart rate is 134 beats per minute. If you go above that heart rate, your body turns on the anaerobic system.

Some additional factors for determining maximum heart rate:

- Add five to your maximum heart rate if you are in excellent health and have been injury free for two years.
- Subtract five from your maximum heart rate if you suffer from chronic health issues or had an injury in the last year.

For example, I'm a 36-year-old with no major injury for the last two years and I have been working out consistently, so my max aerobic fitness heart rate is 149 (180-36 +5).

So, when I'm doing my movements (running, swimming, kayaking, hiking, lifting, etc.), I work to keep my heart rate between 139 and 149 beats per minute. This way, I'm getting the most out of exercising without stressing my adrenals or burning sugar.

Lastly, and possibly most importantly, make sure you warm up and cool down after exercise. This should be at least 10 minutes of moving to slowly warm up and cool down your body. A proper warm-up allows your heart rate and blood flow to slowly adjust.

THE M.A.F. TEST

Dr. Phil Maffatone, who happens to be one of my favorite doctors and authors, describes the M.A.F. test in his writings. He say M.A.F. stands for **Maximum Aerobic Function**, although I think that perhaps **Mitochondrial Assessment of Function** might be a better name, as what it really measures is the efficiency of energy production from the mitochondria.

The test is simple. Just go for a run, walk, bike, row, etc. at your maximum aerobic heart rate and time it. Go for 30 minutes and measure the distance you went. The more efficient your oxygen burning mitochondria are, the farther you will be able to go in the 30 minute period. It's best to do this in a controlled space like a home treadmill or gym so all other factors remain the same.

I strongly encourage you to do this, as tracking your improvement is a wonderful way to stay motivated. By performing this test monthly, you can measure how your mitochondria progressively improve function. If all of a sudden your numbers start dropping, something in your life is stressing you, and you should either rest more or find what stresses need to be removed from you life.

It's that simple!

CONCLUSIONS TO THE AIR ELEMENT

- Add more plants to your home or move to nature.
- Perform your diaphragm stretches and Oxygen Flush Breathing daily, ideally first thing in the morning.
- Do at least 10,000 movements per day.
- Before exercising, perform Ragland's test to make sure your able. If necessary, supplement your weakened adrenals and heart.
- When you exercise, make sure you stay below your max aerobic heart rate and monitor your improvement monthly with the M.A.F. Test.

So now that you got your got your air back again, you can move on to the amazing characteristics of living water!

19 WATER SAFETY

ELEMENT—WATER

Many years from now, I believe researches will look back on American society, much like Roman society, and know that part of our downfall was due to poisoned water. The Romans were poisoned by lead in their water. They used lead pipes in transporting water and lead pots for making their wine. Romans loved their wine and they found that if they simmered grapes in lead pots it made the wine sweeter and allowed it to last longer. This is where lead first got its reputation as "the sweet poison." The Romans' consumption of copious amounts of wine spiked by sweet poison contributed to the downfall of their society. America's copious consumption of city water and non-structured water is leading many of us to our own Roman-style breakdown.

The issue of potable water is a priority in the world today, and for good reason, but not the reasons I'm going to discuss in this chapter. While we are running out of fresh water reserves, what I'm going to discuss is the importance of water to human health. In this chapter, you will learn how living, structured water in the correct amounts can literally reprogram our bodies, charge our cells and regenerate diseased tissue. You will also learn how dead, unstructured water will shut down our enzyme systems, lower our IQ, create arthritis, sap our cells of energy and rapidly age us. Unknowingly, most of us are consuming this zombie dead water and with it creating devastating health issues.

We live on the water planet and we are a water body. Water covers approximately 70% of the planet, which fittingly is the same percentage of water in the human body. In essence, our bodies are just a bag full of electrically charged water-filled cells, floating in a water-driven lymphatic system and surrounded by a watery bag of skin.

Many physicians say, "we're not sick, we're thirsty." The great sages of the past believed water is the connection between the substantial (body) and substantive (spirit) world. The Bible begins by saying, "God moved upon the spirit of the water" and ends by saying, "And let him that is thirsty come. And whosoever will, let him take the water of life freely." References to healing waters are made in every religion of the world. These words will take on new meaning after you read this chapter and begin to understand the properties of water.

The really fascinating thing about water is how crystal formations are created when water molecules interact. These formations can store and pass on vast quantities of information from our outside environment inward. The body uses this information for movement of fluids, healing, delivering energy to tissues, signaling our cellular environment, and much, much more. If our bodies were computers (which they essentially are), water would be the operating system. If we consume the wrong water it's like programming our body with malware. The right type of water has a molecular structure naturally imbibed with order and intelligence, and when consumed will increase the body's ability to heal.

To align ourselves with the water element, we must first make sure that we're not poisoning ourselves by drinking dead water spiked with pollutants, heavy metals and chemicals. The second step is to learn how to find and consume energized, structured, and living water. Accomplish this in two steps:

STEP ONE—REMOVE TOXIC WATER

According to the *New York Times* one in five Americans drink tap water polluted from contaminates, and they estimate that since 2004 50 million Americans have been contaminated.[93] *USA Today* agrees, stating that 4 million Americans per year are exposed to unhealthy drinking water.[94] The problem is widespread and expanding faster than ever. Many Americans are showing the *obvious* symptoms of consuming poor water (think Flint, Michigan), but I would argue the amount being negatively affected by water is closer to 90%. You'll soon see why I say this.

While it's not necessary for you to understand *every* chemical in tap water that can harm us, as the list is very long, it is important to understand a few. Among the worst are agricultural runoff, chlorine and fluoride. Here is a short explanation of some of the major contributors to poisoned water in America:

AGRICULTURAL RUNOFF

With the advent of modern agriculture and GMO foods, the use of chemicals has increased exponentially. Unfortunately, all these petroleum- and nitrogen-based chemicals don't just disappear, but run off into the groundwater, streams, rivers and oceans. Research has proven that over time it is accumulating by a multiple of ten every 10-20 years.[95] This accumulation of widespread agricultural pollution is known as non-point water pollution because it doesn't come from a single source. It's everywhere.

These pollutants have become so bad that there are frequent harmful algae blooms (HABs) occurring all over the USA. The pollutants work by blocking the oxygen, killing the marine life, and producing harmful toxins. Last year in my home state, we had algae blooms in both Lake Erie and the Ohio River. According to the Environmental Protection Agency, these blooms are happening in all 50 states. They produce dead zones in water bodies where no life can survive. There is currently a dead zone in the Gulf of Mexico over 6,000 square miles, all originating from toxins coming down the Mississippi. Think about that for a second.

In 2008, the U.S. government created a report called "Harmful Algae Bloom (HABS) Management and Response: Assessment and Plan." The report warned, "It is widely believed that the frequency and geographic distribution of HABs have been increasing worldwide. All U.S. coastal states have experienced HABs over the last decade, and new species have emerged in some locations that were not previously known to cause problems."[96]

This agricultural pollution affects all levels of wildlife and the environment, and since we sit on the top of the food chain, it affects us significantly. The greatest concern from all these pollutants is how they affect the human endocrine system as "endocrine disrupters." These act on the endocrine system by mimicking natural hormones and create a range of health issues including lowered sperm count, sexual birth defects, and cancer of sex organs.

Cities and the EPA, in an effort to provide clean drinking water, use a progressively growing list of chemicals in an attempt to clean it, yet they frequent fall short. According to the EPA, it's impossible for cities and municipalities to remove all harmful chemicals so instead they publish a list called (CCL) Contaminate Candidate List of the chemicals that are still in the water. This list is updated every five years. Most municipalities can only monitor many of the chemicals in the water and attempt to keep them at "acceptable" levels by adding new chemicals. The worst amongst these are chlorine and fluoride.

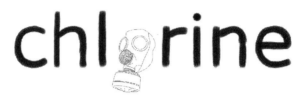

"Chlorine is the greatest crippler and killer of modern times. It is an insidious poison." —Dr. Joseph M. Price, MD, Moseby's Medical Dictionary

The main focus of municipal water systems is to eliminate algae, bacteria, fungus and parasites. To do this, most use chlorine as a method of killing. Chlorine gas is created by putting an electrical current through salt water. It was first used in World War I as a way of poisoning the enemy, and after the war found its way into our water supply with detrimental health effects. By compressing the gas to a liquid they found a way to transport it and add it to water supplies. When added to water, chlorine creates a compound that is similar to a diluted bleach. Like any medication that kills bacteria, it has prevented some waterborne diseases but certainly replaced them with new diseases of modern commerce. Soon after World War I, with the additional of chlorination, incidences of cancer, organ disease, immune disorders, neurological disorders, hardening of the arteries, and birth defects skyrocketed.

When chlorine is added to water, it forms Trihalomethanes (THMs), one of which is chloroform. The U.S. Council of Environmental Quality states,

"Cancer risk among people using chlorinated water is as much as 93 percent higher than among those whose water does not contain chlorine."[97]

BreastCancerFund.org states, "Long-term drinking of chlorinated water appears to increase a person's risk of developing bladder cancer by as much as 80% ... and ... one common factor among women with breast cancer is that they all have 50 to 60% higher levels of chlorination byproducts (THMs) in their fat tissue than women without breast cancer..."[98] A three year long Norwegian study of 141,000 child births found a 14% increased risk of birth defects in areas with chlorinated water.[99]

No! Say it can't be! Skyrocketing disease and putting poison in the water is just a coincidence, right? Without a doubt it adds to the cumulative allostatic stress on our bodies and should be avoided if at all possible.

Thankfully, chlorine is easy to filter out of the water and almost all activated carbon filters remove the majority of it. But you know what isn't easy to filter out of water?

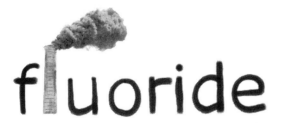

"We would not purposely add arsenic to the water supply. And we would not purposely add lead. But we do add fluoride. The fact is that fluoride is more toxic than lead and just slightly less toxic than arsenic." —Dr. John Yiamouyiannis

In 1939, a man named Henry Trendley Dean, now called "The Father of Fluoridation," studied teeth of 15,000 children in 272 cities where *natural fluoride* occurred. He then presented data on 21 cities that indicated that *natural fluoride* reduced cavities. Later he admitted twice in court that his reports were flawed and they did not support fluoridation.[100] However, the die was cast and the fluoride movement had begun.

Through a well-organized campaign, the belief that sodium fluoride (which is not the same as **natural potassium fluoride**) hardens teeth quickly spread. Sodium fluoride is not a naturally occurring substance, but rather a *toxic byproduct literally scraped from the smoke stacks of the phosphate fertilizer industry*. Not only did the fertilizer industry no longer have to pay for proper disposal of a toxic pollutant, but they began to make a profit by selling this to municipal water suppliers.

Based on Henry Dean's theories, sodium fluoride was added to municipal water supplies starting in 1945 in Grand Rapids, Michigan as an experimental city. Muskegon, Michigan was the control city to see if there were any differences in health occurring between the two. Unfortunately before any results were gathered, sodium fluoride was added to municipalities all over the country. Even the control city of Muskegon began adding fluoride to its water in 1951. In response to the widespread use, the European commission stated "There is no tissue or cellular process that requires fluoride".[101]

The belief evolved that fluoride is a nutrient required for healthy strong teeth, and that a deficiency

226

of fluoride leads to cavities. However, fluoride is not a nutrient and the FDA does not list it as an essential element. The British Medical Journal has stated that "Fluoride is not in any natural metabolic pathways"[102] and even the CDC states that fluoride content of teeth has little bearing on whether a tooth will develop a cavity.[103]

To this day, there is *no evidence* that we are protecting teeth with sodium fluoride in our water. The National Institute of Dental Research did a study in 1990, the largest to date, on 39,000 children in over 84 cities at a cost of $4 million. The result was that there was *no* statistical difference in tooth decay in fluoridated and non-fluoridated communities.[104] Further proof showing the ineffectiveness of fluoride comes from four cities in four different countries (Cuba, Finland, Germany, Canada) that dropped water fluoridation and found no statistical increase in cavities.[105]

Worse still than the fact that fluoride doesn't work and is not a natural ingredient in the body is that it's incredibly toxic to humans. Nobel Prize winner Dr. James Sumner stated in 1958, "We ought to go slowly. Everybody knows that fluorides are very poisonous substances... We use them in enzyme chemistry to poison enzymes, those vital agents in the body. That is the reason things are poisoned; because the enzymes are poisoned and that is why animals and plants die." Robert Carton, a Ph.D. and former EPA scientist once said, "fluoridation is the greatest case of scientific fraud of this century, if not all time." *Time* magazine on April 12, 2010, included fluoride in its "Top Ten Common Household Toxins."

In a recent interview, I asked a chemist named Ron Greinke what would happen if I ate an entire tube of fluoridated toothpaste. He told me that it would kill me.

He went on to explain that fluoride is more toxic than lead and a dose of five grams is lethal and even at the nanogram level shuts down 62 different enzyme systems in the body. The Journal of the Canadian Dental Association states "fluoride supplements should not be recommended for children less than 3 years old."[106]

The real problem arises from the fact fluoride has a long half life and, accumulated in our bodies, can create fluoridosis of the teeth (white spots) and bones, arthritis, phantom pains, and fractures in the body. Three studies in the Journal of American Medical Association showed links between hip fractures and fluoride.[107],[108],[109]

Sodium fluoride has been proven to lower IQ. The Harvard School of Public Health posted a systematic review of 27 published studies on IQ on more than 8,000 children and reported on it in *Environmental Health Perspectives* on July 20, 2012. Senior researcher Philippe Grandjean stated, "fluoride seems to fit in with lead, mercury and other poisons that can cause chemical brain drain. The effects of each toxicant may seem small, but the combined damage on a population scale can be serious, especially because the brain power of the next generation is crucial to all of us." The study showed that, on average, drinking fluoride water lowers IQ by seven points.

So why in the world are we putting this in our water? Why are the drinking fountains in our schools spiked with this toxin? Their answer: "Don't worry about it, look the other way, move along, nothing to see here." That's because someone is making a ton of money. Seriously? Moral of the story: Don't trust the government with your health and *don't drink their water* without cleaning out the toxins.

HOW TO CLEAN WATER

Tap water created by municipalities is not fit for human consumption. The sources of water for consumption should be spring water from a clean aquifer, well water, distilled water, or reverse osmosis (RO) water. There are endless debates about the benefits and characteristics of the varying sources. Some physicians believe distilled water is therapeutic, as it's completely empty of everything, including minerals. Since it's empty, it will leech minerals from the body. At times, this can be beneficial because most people have an accumulation of indigestible inorganic calcium within their arteries. I believe that distilled water should be used only during a fast or detoxification period.

Most experts I speak with believe that reverse osmosis is the best filtration system as it removes all chemicals (including agricultural runoff, fluoride, and chlorine) and organisms such as bacteria and parasites. These filters require maintenance, so follow installation and maintenance directions.

Well water and spring water should be regularly checked for pollutants, chemicals, live organisms and all other health hazards. If possible, it's ideal to consume water directly from a spring, especially if you know the source or trust the company acquiring the spring water.

The reality for most of us is that a good filtration or reverse osmosis system must be purchased and can be done so for several hundred dollars. Make no excuses, go out today and purchase a quality unit or move to a place with clean water. Once you have the poison out, the next step it to ensure that the water is living and structured.

20 - LIVING, STRUCTURED WATER

ELEMENT—WATER

Anyone who wants more energy and a supercharged body should be deeply fascinated in the concept of structured water. All water has polarized hydrogen atoms that are slightly attracted to each other. You can see this with water when two drops quickly become one when they touch. Because of this attraction water molecules can combine in an infinite number of ways, creating geometric patterns at the molecular level. Structured water can be frozen and the patterns can be observed, as anyone who has ever looked at a snowflake knows.

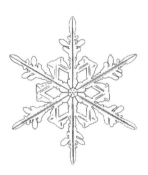

When water is charged with energy, it will form into a structured hexagonal liquid crystalline formation and is known as living water. This living water can hold a great deal of information via frequencies. Water picks up frequencies of what's around it and holds onto them, imprinting that energy into the structure of the water based on how the hydrogen atoms attract and interact with each other.

Water that is polluted, stagnant, or without minerals loses its energy. The hydrogen bonds break and re-form rapidly in random, non-structured ways. This is dead water. Even if this water is cleaned and filtered to remove the pollution, it cannot re-structure or re-mineralize itself. This dead water does little to hydrate the body or charge the cells.

Nature has plenty of methods to perfectly structure water. Our planet has the North and South Poles, which naturally create order within water. As water is filtered through the layers of the planet, it is naturally cleansed by carbon and rock and picks up mineral and salt imprints. As water moves through the planet, it gains energy. As the water matures it naturally comes up to the surface in the form of springs, where it begins to move. As it moves through streams, it conforms to whatever it encounters. This movement energizes the water. In nature, it runs over the ground, down streams, over waterfalls, goes into lakes and oceans. The moon creates tides and currents, sloshing the oceans back and forth and further building its energy. The sun evaporates the water and drops it back onto the earth with precipitation, but always water is moving. As soon as it becomes stagnant it quickly becomes diseased.

When water moves, it can become highly energized from naturally occurring water vortices. A vortex is a swirling of the water. These vortices are found in streams, weather patterns and the ocean. It can be seen as water drains out of sink, or bubbles up underneath a waterfall. It can be see in a water spout, a tornado, motion of the clouds around a hurricane, or the shape of the waves moving over a reef. Animal life frequently accumulates in places where natural vortices occur in water. Salmon jumping up waterfalls to get to their spawning grounds do so with the help of energy from vortices. Trout can swim stationary with almost no expenditure of energy by swimming within the natural occurring vortices in a stream. In the ocean, krill and small fish accumulate in these vortices, which attracts all levels of marine life. Many shells of wildlife, such as snails, have the spiral vortex imprinted on them.

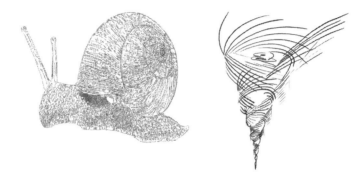

This movement of energy imbibes the oxygen and hydrogen into an organized, hexagonal, crystalline structure. All vortices or spirals conform to a ratio found frequently in nature known as the Fibonacci golden sequence.

Water that is polluted with chemicals or forced to sit stationary without movement quickly denigrates into unstructured forms. The flowing of water through straight pipes, as it does in our homes, does not structure it. Additionally, once streams are straightened and the water loses its structure, the presence of wildlife quickly diminishes.

The seminal book *Hidden Messages in the Water* by Masaru Emoto, Ph.D. showed what happens to water that has been quickly crystallized after exposure to a variety of different levels of stimuli. A dark field microscope revealed the incredible crystalline beauty of natural waters from some of the world's cleanest sources. Water that had been exposed to classical music such as Chopin and Bach was also highly structured, symmetrical, and beautiful. On the flip side, crystals from water from polluted sources or exposed to hateful music showed random, non-symmetrical crystals. When water is exposed to angry hateful words like, "you make me sick, I will kill you," it forms into twisted, random and non-symmetrical patterns. What he was able to show through this experimentation is that water holds onto energy patterns that it's exposed to.

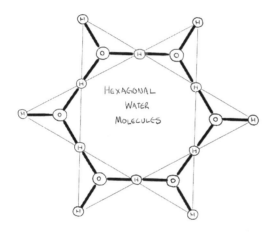

STRUCTURED WATER IN THE BODY

In the 30 years since Dr. Mu Shirk Jhon first presented his theories on aging in his book *Molecular Water Environment*, we have known that aging is created in large part by the loss of structured, energized water from our cells. He showed that healthy DNA is surrounded by highly structured crystalline water and is necessary for proper expression.

As water becomes more structured, it becomes more dense and represents a majority of our intracellular water. A healthy person should have 60% of their total water inside their cells and 40% outside in the lymph, blood and extracellular environment. This ratio is ideal for cellular function. As people lose water from their cells, their skin wrinkles, their height shrinks and their cellular energy plummets. The process of losing intracellular water is the process of dying. The more we resist it, the more we resist and delay death itself.

When people drink unstructured, polluted, low mineral water, it quickly depletes their life energy and changes DNA expression. It's not taken up well by the cells and dehydrates our internal cellular environment. The most common symptoms that people complain of when this happens is a loss of energy. When I measure people in my office, I always find a correlation of low intracellular water to low cellular charge and low energy. To correct their energy and the low intracellular water, I have them quit sugar, take minerals and enzymes, increase the oxygen in the their bodies, and drink remineralized, structured water.

HOW THE HEART STRUCTURES WATER

In a beautiful book called *Human Heart, Cosmic Heart,* Cardiologist Thomas Cowen, M.D. paints a picture of how the heart functions that will surprise most people. He posits and proves with models, charts and studies that the human heart is not a pump but acts more like a hydraulic dam. He makes the argument that blood moving through the body does so more by a hydrophilic mechanism than by the movement of a pump, as the current theory how the heart functions now suggests. This hydrophilic motion is similar to how water moves up a tree or is pulled through a siphon. Cowen states that this movement is generated by a layer of structured water within the arteries that creates an electrical charge that propels the forward motion of blood. He argues that if blood moved from a heart pumping action, the red blood cells in the capillaries would not be able to stop and start up again. He says in his book: "What's amazing is that blood actually stops moving in the capillaries, which is necessary for the efficient exchange of gases, nutrients, and waste products. After the blood stops moving, it oscillates slightly, and then begins to flow again as it enters the veins." He goes on to ask the obvious question, "So if the function of the heart is not a pump, then what is it for?" He goes on to state that the function of the heart beating is to create vortices as the blood sloshes through the chambers of the heart. These vortices create the structured water that lines our blood vessels, propelling our blood forward and nourishing all the cells of the body.

The current theory of heart disease states that blockages in the arteries that shut off oxygen supply to the heart are what cause angina and then heart attacks. This theory has been disproven through studies that have shown that the body's oxygen levels do not change during a heart attack.[110]

Cowen documents that 80% of heart events are preceded by deficits in the parasympathetic system created by too much chronic allostatic stress. Studies show that heart attacks result when the parasympathetic nervous system is reduced by more than a third. Chronic stress reduces our nutritional reserves and lowers the electrical charge throughout the body. The body will sacrifice every tissue in the body in an effort to preserve cardiac function but when the level of stress and resulting decrease in the parasympathetic system reach a tipping point, the electrical charge lowers within the arteries. This creates areas where "unstructured" exclusion zones occur. The body's response to these exclusion zones is to create inflammation and lay down a calcium cast to support these weakened zones. This, of course, turns into plaque.

Cowen suggests that to cure heart disease (and all other disease), we must protect our parasympathetic system by reducing stress. He says that to do this we must learn to live in a manner quite different than the norms of the industrial civilization of which we are a part. In short, we must nourish our bodies. How? First, by removing stressors such as sugar, emotional stress, and toxic water. Then, by adding in things that fill us up. Things like healthy relationships, self-love, and a low carbohydrate diet rich in minerals and fats. Cowen states that one way of massively reducing the stress that drains our electrical energy is to quit drinking toxic, unstructured tap water. Instead, we should only be consuming structured, mineralized, high-energy water that can support all levels of cellular function. As we do this, the parasympathetic nervous system will rebound, heart function will re-establish, and the re-formation of structured water within the exclusion zones will ensue. Thus, healing will occur.

Heart disease was practically unheard of 100 years ago and today it kills more than 700,000 people annually in the USA. Most people did not drink tap water one hundred years ago. Is it possible that the process of creating unstructured water spiked with chlorine and fluoride and distributing it via a central sewer and water distribution network is reducing the structuring water throughout our bodies? Is it possible this change in our water lowers our cellular energy and increases all levels of modern disease including heart disease? The obvious answer is *yes*.

STRUCTURING WATER

There are many ways to give water energy, but before it can be charged two things must happen. It first needs to be free of toxic chemicals and then there must be some minerals in the water to hold the charge. Only then can water respond to organizing energy. There are many suggestions out there on how to imbibe water with energy. Some people believe that putting crystals in the water can energize it. Emoto showed that simply writing the words "I love you" on a water bottle or by exposing the water to beautiful music will structure it. Emoto also showed that praying or blessing the water energizes it. This belief underlies the basis of baptism and holy water. Since water holds the energy it's exposed to, whatever is done to the water will imprint it. A powerful way to energize water seems to be by moving it in a spiral vortex, and this is the technique I use. I suggest you use as many as you are able. For ideas on structuring and further leaning into this topic, read the book *Dancing with Water* written by MJ Pangman & Malante Evans.

Do not ever drink or cook with municipal tap water, and try not to drink water out of plastic bottles. Instead, drink spring water delivered to your house or purchased from a health food store, preferably in glass containers, or clean the municipal water with an RO filter. Then, take the water through a two step process:

1.) Add a small amount of real salt (Celtic, Himalayan, etc.) to the water to remineralize it.
2.) Energize the water. The most effective machine I've encountered for this is called a water vitalizer. A water vitalizer looks similar to a blender and, when turned on, creates a vortex in the water by spinning it rapidly for 8-26 minutes. Once it's structured, it should be refrigerated since cold water better maintains structured energy. When

you leave the house, take your own water with you
wherever you go in a glass or metal water bottle.

Conclusion of the Water element:
For the next 21 days, and preferably for life, drink
only clean and structured water.

21 - SUNS HEALING FIRE

ELEMENT—FIRE

"Keep your face always toward the sunshine, and shadows will fall behind you." —Walt Disney

If you walk yourself through the Whole Body Health reset and prepare yourself to be ignited, the therapies discussed in the FIRE element will create a health explosion. This is why I've saved the element of fire for the end of the book. If you have not prepared yourself to be activated, then the flame of healing will not spread.

The three characteristics of the energy or FIRE element in the body are: first, increase your exposure to external sources of energy via the sun. Next, improve the transmission of that energy through your body through chiropractic care. Finally employ cannabis oil to stimulate new healthy cells that can maintain the charge. While there are literally thousands of examples of how to do each of these steps, I have identified and extensively tested three of the most powerful and effective and will discuss how to use these therapies to recharge your cellular batteries.

Three aspects of FIRE element on the body

- The Sun—the source of all energy on Earth
- The nervous system—how we transmit the charge to every cell in our body
- Powerful medicine—cannabis to help the cells to take up the charge

THE SUN

The sun is the source of all energy on Earth. The sun
warms the planet, plant life converts the sun's rays
through photosynthesis to energy, animals eat those
plants and gain their energy. Some of us, in turn, eat
animals and gain their energy. Coal and oil are nothing
more than ancient deposits of plants that were
concentrated into energy over millions of years. All
energy on Earth and within our bodies can be traced
back to the power of the sun. Everything lives and dies
as a direct result of gaining or losing the sun's energy.

Perhaps this is why every past great civilization on
earth believed that the sun possessed supernatural
powers. The Aztecs, Mayans, and Incas built temples to
the sun. The Ancient Egyptians believed that the
Pharaoh was the sun's representative on Earth and built
pyramids in honor of the sun. The Hindu tradition
spoke frequently of the healing powers the sun provides.
Native Americans built monuments and had rituals
around the sun. Even the ancient Europeans built
monumental stone structures honoring the sun. Every
successful culture honored the sun and for the most part
had far better health than we enjoy today. Perhaps there
is a lesson to be learned by those civilizations that came
before us.

Even the religion of modern medicine is now gaga
over the sun in the form of vitamin D. Vitamin D is one
of the compounds that increases in our bodies when
we're exposed to the sun. For the last 40 years, science
has known that there is an inverse relationship between
sun exposure and cancer. Re-read that last sentence 10
times. There is an inverse relationship between sun
exposure and cancer. The only cancer that increases with

too much sun exposure is skin cancer, yet 95% of skin cancer is not life threatening.[111]

And yet we are repeatedly told to avoid the sun. Wear sunglasses! Slather on sunblock! But why?

Dr. Weston A. Price, in his historic book *Nutrition and Physical Degeneration* said, "A question arises as to the efficiency of the human body in removing all of the minerals from the ingested foods. Extensive laboratory determinations have shown that most people cannot absorb more than half of the calcium and phosphorus from the foods eaten. The amounts utilized depend directly on the presence of other substances, particularly fat-soluble vitamins."

Thanks to Price, we now know that the body requires fat-soluble vitamin D in order to utilize and absorb minerals. Without sufficient vitamin D, our cells cannot efficiently take up minerals. Since minerals are how our cells hold their cellular charge, without sufficient vitamin D our cells quickly lose their charge.

When the human body needs to send or store electricity, it accomplishes the task via metals and minerals—copper, lithium, trace minerals, etc. Without the sun, we cannot utilize the minerals in the foods we eat, without sufficient minerals the vitamins have little function in the body. Without vitamins our cells have no function. Without function we lose cellular energy and quickly become ill.

A few studies to further illustrate:

  ○ Harvard Medical School published a study in the journal *Circulation* in 2008 that showed that people with very low vitamin D levels (below 10 ng/ml) had an 80% increase in heart disease compared with those with a Vitamin D level above 15 ng/ml. We now know that optimal vitamin D levels are above 60 ng/ml. Americans spend more than $400 billion per year fighting heart disease. How much could be saved if we simply focused on the getting more sun?

° A 2004 study of 187,000 people by the Harvard School of Public Health spanning 21 years in 2004 showed that women who had a vitamin D level over 39 ng/ml were 62% less likely to develop multiple sclerosis than those with the lowest level.

° Studies have shown that 25% of breast cancers have been linked to insufficient sunlight.[112]

° Vitamin D and Alzheimer's disease have been linked. *Science Daily* published a six-year study showing that people who are vitamin D deficient were more than twice as likely to develop dementia and Alzheimer's disease. [113]

A physician named John Tilden once said that if you have the ability to heal even one condition, you have the ability to heal any condition as the process of healing always invokes the same principle. So what is your cellular health?

The results are very clear. Most people are very deficient in vitamin D and have low cellular charge. Therefore, most people need more access to the sun and, by definition, more vitamin D. There are three ways of getting more sun and the Whole Body Health Warrior should consider all three:

1. Get more sunshine on your skin.
2. Get more sunlight in your eyes.
3. Consume stored sunlight in the form of vitamin D and animal fat.

1. Get more sunshine on your skin.

The way that our bodies produce vitamin D is from UVB rays directly hitting our skin. The UVB rays are present in most parts of the world only between 10 a.m. and 2 p.m. and only during the summer months. The goal should be to get as much sunshine as we're able during these times until we get lightly pink, without any feelings of burning on the skin. The only way we get damaged skin and most skin cancers is if we repeatedly burn our skin.

The critic might say that this destroys your skin after years of chronic exposure, and they are partly right. But by using coconut oil on our skin after sun exposure we can avoid most detrimental effects that chronic sun exposure pose. Wrinkles are created by the drying out of the skin from the sun, so by keeping properly hydrated (structured water) and our skin nourished (coconut oil), we can avoid most of the skin-damaging effects.

Many people ignorantly put on highly toxic sunscreen that blocks the UVB rays, yet allows in many of the UVA rays. According to the American Cancer Society, UVA rays are more highly associated with skin cancer.[114] Therefore, it makes little sense to ever wear sunscreen. If you find yourself in a situation where you know your skin is going to burn because you're spending the entire day at the beach or on a boat, it is best to protect your skin with a hat and clothing. If you still feel the need to use sunscreen, then use natural zinc oxide sunscreen. This is not the sexy coconut smelling spray that immediately disappears on your skin, but rather the dorky white stuff that never fully disappears that many of us remember our mothers applying liberally when we were little.

Since many of us live in a place with a winter, or simply don't have the time or ability to spend too much time out in the sun, the use of tanning beds becomes necessary. There are "safe" tanning beds. When going to a tanning salon, ask which bed has the highest UVB rays. Doing this once per week is often enough to raise vitamin D levels to an acceptable level.

2. Get more sunlight directly in your eyes.

Almost all healthy aspects of nature need to be taken as the whole to get the entire benefit. Medicine always seeks the active and usually patentable ingredient while ignoring the whole. One specific example is aspirin, which is one ingredient of white willow bark. White willow bark provides highly effective pain relief with literally no side effects. Yet when you take just the active ingredient out—aspirin—it causes bleeding of the stomach. The examples of unintended pharmaceutical effects are endless and well-documented in countless class-action lawsuits.

The sun is no different. When we try to extrapolate that the only benefit of the sun is Vitamin D and then seek to reproduce a synthetic high dose version, the benefits pale in comparison to the actual source. The ingredient that most people never think about when it comes to the sun is how we need the exposure in our eyes.

Our eyes? "But I was told that UV rays in the eyes cause damage so I've always worn sunglasses to protect them," you might say. Looking at the sun during the peak hours of UV rays will of course cause damage, which is why we don't look directly at the sun during these hours.

Sunlight into the eyes has been shown to stimulate healthy hormone function in the body. According to a

2008 study in the *British Journal of Ophthalmology* photoreceptors in the eyes play a vital role in human physiology and health.

Again, the ancients had this figured out. Many successful cultures practiced sun gazing. I first heard about sun gazing a few years ago while in Central America. There is a growing practice of looking directly into the sun for the first 30 minutes of the morning and the last 30 minutes of the day. Have you ever wondered why humans are naturally drawn to watch sunrises and sunsets? We don't know why but it naturally feels good.

Native Americans, Hindi, and many other cultures had a tradition of looking directly into the sun during the first and last 30 minutes of the day. It was believed to have highly meditative effects, refueling one's body and soul while ridding it of impurities. Some cultures believed that looking into "heaven's eye" opens a connection to the supernatural and elevated the viewer's wellbeing.

This age-old practice of sun gazing has been rediscovered around the world and many cultures, retreat centers, and holistic healers are using it effectively to stimulate the bodies energy to be activated.

It's now documented scientific fact that there exists a direct connection between the eye's photoreceptors and hormonal health. In 1972, a doctor named Robert Moore first traced the pathway of light through the body by means of radioactive material. He found that the light went from retinal neurons to clusters of neurons deep in the hypothalamus called the Suprachiasmiatic Nuclei (SCN cells). For the next several decades, Moore and other researchers investigated the purpose of these SCN cells. They found that these cells are central to the secretion of "most if not all the major hormones and neurotransmitters

245

within the body."[115] Over the following years, Moore discovered that these SCN cells exist throughout the entire body and most especially within our endocrine glands and major organs. These cells synchronize with light, directing the functionality of our metabolism and how our body responds to stress. An effective way of activating these SCN cells and our hormonal response is to gaze directly into the sun during the "safe" hours of the morning and evening.

My own observation is that the hormone system is always the last thing to fail before health drops. No one ever comes into my clinic with chronic illness until their hormone system has failed—this is phase III of exhaustion. This failure is always directly connected to exposure to chronic stress and the loss of cellular charge.

While no single activity is a cure-all, sun exposure for both the skin and eyes is a key factor of any effective health protocol.

HOW TO SUN GAZE

Why do we watch the sunrise? Why do we concentrate on it? In order to learn to mobilize all our thoughts, all our desires, and all our energies, and to direct them toward the realization of the highest ideal. A person who works to unify the many chaotic forces that pull him in every direction and to project them in a single, luminous and salutary direction becomes such a powerful center that his presence, like the sun, is able to radiate through space. Yes, he who manages to control the tendencies of his lower nature can spread these blessings over the whole of humanity, and he becomes a sun. He lives in such freedom that he expands the field of his consciousness to include the entire human race, to which he sends the abundance of light and love that pour forth from him. —Omraam Mikhaël Aïvanhov

246

First begin by attempting to look at the sun for 30 seconds at a time during the first and last 30 minutes of the day. As you're able, work up to 30 second intervals. After these intervals, put your hands over your eyes and look away from the sun as your vision normalizes. Work up to a full 30 minutes of sun gazing while watching the sunrise and sunset. My clinical view is that the benefits of this activity are due to the activation of the photoreceptors in the eyes, but I think we all know the benefits of quietly watching a sunset go beyond explanation.

Many have reported that their vision improves with daily sun gazing. Some have reported that after incorporating sun gazing regularity they feel less hunger and need less food, as the sun provides direct energy to the cells. The only practice to date that definitively lengthens life is consuming less calories.[116] To my great disbelief, I have met people that eat almost no food and claim that their energy and often long-life comes from deep breathing (as described in the air element chapters) and from the practice of sun gazing.

WARNING:

Looking directly into the sun can cause eye damage. This is no different than the damage caused by sitting too close to a fire. We all have a different sensitivity to light, so please practice caution and start conservatively when sun gazing. Going out and trying to stare directly into the sun for 20 minutes on your first try is folly. Practice common sense when increasing your sun exposure.

CONSUMING STORED SUNLIGHT

The bodies of all animals store sunlight in the form of fat that is most concentrated in the liver. It therefore makes obvious sense that consuming liver and animal fat is an excellent source of fat-soluble vitamins, which include vitamin D and therefore stored sunlight. This is one of the reasons that Cod Liver Oil has always been considered one of the most nutrient-dense superfoods. By consuming it and other forms of animal fat, people living in the Arctic who get very little sunlight still have normal vitamin D levels and are capable of vibrant health.

A vast quantity of research has shown that healthy animal fat does not cause heart disease and is a necessary building block of the human body. Fats forms the basis of our cell walls, our hormones, our nervous system, and brain. Most of these cannot be replicated in the body, which is why they are called "Essential Fatty Acids." Since most energy is derived in the body from sugar or fat, and since we seek to eliminate sugar, it becomes necessary to consume more fat. When consuming fat, the quality of the fat is of the utmost importance. Fat is essentially concentrated energy, so if we consume oxidized fats spiked with hormones, antibiotics, and toxins, it will quickly damage our bodies.

Any animal that consumes green plant life will collect vitamin D in its fat and liver, and this animal's flesh will provide a much healthier source of fat. Animals in feed operations consuming soy, corn, grain, cottonseed, etc. have few fat-soluble vitamins. Therefore, grass-fed beef contains much more vitamin D than farm-raised fish. Make sense? So when we consume animal fat it becomes imperative that we carefully consider how our food was raised. I try to never consume animals from feed operations, as I know they are devoid of necessary nutrients. It also bears mention that Confined Animal Feed Operations (CAFO) are akin to animal abuse.

When seeking to supplement vitamin D, we need to understand a couple of things. First, it's best to get it from a whole food source whenever possible. The foods containing the highest levels of vitamin D are liver followed by grass-fed butter, egg yolks and fat wild-caught fish. You can usually recognize the fats that are high in fat-soluble vitamins because of the slightly orange coloring. This color is created by the fat-soluble vitamin A, which is congruently found with Vitamin D. People will recognize this color if you've ever seen grass-fed butter like Kerrygold along side industrial white butter.

Taking vitamin D in supplement form is always derived from some animal source, and it's very important that it be emulsified in fat for absorption. I have seen so many people with low vitamin D levels go to their doctor and get a vitamin D prescription with very little improvement in their blood work and health. When given a whole food vitamin D emulsified in fat, their blood levels quickly normalize.

HOW MUCH TO CONSUME

It's very important that we measure our vitamin D levels yearly, as it should stay within an ideal range of 60-100 ng/ml. The problems associated with too low a level are more wide-ranging and dangerous than too much. If you are unsure, consider increasing the dose. While overdosing can cause toxicity and organ damage to occur, I have never seen our recommended dose result in toxicity. That usually occurs when taking prescription doses of 50,000 IUs or more.

If your vitamin D level is less than 15 ng/ml, begin by taking 15,000 IUs per day and six capsules of EPA/DHA. After three months, recheck and if it's above 15 ng/ml, proceed to lower it to 8,000 IUs per day and four capsules of EPA/DHA. Stay at this level until you get up to a blood level of 60 ng/ml. Once you are at or above 60, lower your vitamin D intake to 4,000 IUs per day and three capsules of EPA/DHA. 4000 IUs per day is how much our body needs just to support daily physiological processes. Less than this daily will lead to deficiency over time. If you begin to spend more time outside, lower you supplementation to 2,000 IUs per day and two capsules of EPA/DHA. This should be rechecked yearly to ensure blood levels stay between 60-100 ng/ml.

22 - THE NERVOUS SYSTEM

ELEMENT—FIRE

"The doctor of the future will give no medicine but will interest his patients in the care of the human frame, in diet, and in the cause and prevention of disease."
—Thomas Edison

Our bodies, like all life forms and all technology, contain an electrical system with circuitry. In your home, energy flows in from the electrical source through the circuit breaker and then to every device in your home. The energy in the body follows the exact same principle. As previously explained, all energy is generated from the sun and eventually converted to cellular energy. That control system for that energy flows from the brain and down our spinal cords to progressively smaller and smaller nerve branches until it reaches every cell in the body. It is transmission behind all movement, all organ function, and all life. It is the universal intelligence flowing through our nervous systems that allows our bodies to function, heal, interact with our environment, and connect at all levels of consciousness.

This complex process occurs through millions of impulses firing every second—back and forth from our environment to our brain, through our autonomic nervous system, and back to our environment. This energy and communication system is what allows billions of cells to synchronize for our systems to operate. It's what allows us to respond to our environmental influences in both a conscious and unconscious manner. It's what allows our five senses to pick up stimuli and power breathing, digestion, heart rate, etc. Any blockage or delay in transmission results in loss of function, weakening of the cellular energy, and eventually tissue damage. If a blockage remains long enough, the damaged tissue passes the tipping point of being able to regenerate—this is disease.

Blockages in the flow of this universal organizing nerve energy occur in our bodies due to the lingering effects of past injuries. A physics principle called Wolf's Law states that changes in tissues are created by past mechanical and environmental changes. Since our bodies are being knocked around constantly, most carry years of detrimental changes in their structure. Most of these injuries occur to our tissues or bones without damaging the flow to our nervous system. This is a fractured bone, a cut in your hand, a cold, a torn muscle from exercise, etc. The body is efficient at directing universal intelligence through the nervous system and autocorrecting the damaged cellular environment. This is the miracle of healing—no drugs or doctors are needed and we all experience it daily.

Frequently, however, the injuries we sustain do affect our nervous system. We sustain a head injury, get whiplash from a car accident, or hurt our spine while lifting improperly. Even the constant stress created by poor posture, sitting too long at a computer, and emotional stress can injure our nervous system. These injuries are recorded within our nervous system and cause circuits to trip. This is very similar to what happens in our homes when we plug too many appliances into one circuit. Flow is disrupted. It's a protective mechanism that occurs to protect the entire electrical system. The same is true in the body. The term that has been applied to circuits tripping within our nervous system and the resulting decreased function of sections of our nervous system is called *subluxation*. Subluxation is a section of our nervous system that is powered down, and this is always accompanied by a misalignment in the skeletal structure and fascia housing in that section of the nervous system.

Both Chinese and Western medicines have established that the powering down connected to structural imbalances results in a disorganization of the energy flow through the body. This disorganization of universal intelligence disrupts the electrical forces of the system. This has been called many things in different cultures. In Chinese medicine it's called a block in the Chi. In Western medicine it is called a block of "Universal Intelligence" or a "Subluxation." Hippocrates referred to it as a diminishing of the "Power of Nature." In Sanskrit it's called a blockage of "Prana." They all mean the same thing.

With these changes, we see progressively lowered function and symptoms. Symptomatic changes take time to express themselves and even more time to become diseased. Groups of cells begin to malfunction after years of lowered cellular charge, lowered oxygen, nutrition and absorption. Disease doesn't just show up one day. Nobody goes to bed healthy and then wakes up the next day with cancer. It takes years for cancer to grow from a cluster of a few cells to a size that is detectable, and often years more for outright disease to occur. The lack of organizing energy eventually reaches a tipping point as a heart quits beating or a cancerous growth blocks a vital function.

During energy blockages, the brain does not fully communicate with tissues and is therefore unable to direct Universal Intelligence to create healing. Most of us do not recognize symptoms for what they are—a warning system telling us a change must be made. Instead, through a million commercials and social engineering, we've been brainwashed to go to our doctor or pharmacy and seek man-made chemicals to block the symptoms our bodies use to speak to us. We block the anxiety, the depression, the allergies, the pain. This inevitably leads to more stress, more dysfunction and more disease.

When subluxations are allowed to remain for years, patterns of weakness show in our posture and movements. This is when chronic subluxations become self-propagating in further subluxation and further weakening of Universal Intelligence. We see this often with people as their forward head posture continues to move forward. A human head weighs around 15 pounds, but for every inch of forward head posture it adds 10 more pounds of pressure to the spine and the muscles holding it. Once the head is 4-5 inches forward, the constant pulling on a person's spine further diminishes the flow of energy. As a result, more symptoms arise as the person's light fades.

In this crisis, desperate people seek help and are faced with a choice. Do we go the route of medication, or do we seek to increase the flow of Universal Intelligence in the body? It's impossible to do both as they are competing paradigms. On our website, we have a free education series (video) called "The Truth about Health." In this series we carefully document what happens when we choose the path of standard medicine. A brief summary is that all drugs have negative side-effects and increase cumulative allostatic stress within the body. According to the *Annals of Internal Medicine* most doctors in America have gotten caught up in a "reward system" around prescribing drugs. Drug companies reward doctors for prescribing more drugs. As a result there is a "prescribing cascade" in which doctors prescribe drugs to relieve effects caused by other drugs. Then, of course, doctors add even more drugs to relieve new side effects from recently prescribed drugs.

254

This continues until death occurs. Garbage in, garbage out.

There is, however, the path less traveled and this is the way of the Whole Body Health Warrior. The methods of correction are called applied kinesiology and chiropractic.

APPLIED KINESIOLOGY

Applied kinesiology is a methodology of muscle testing to determine which circuits within the body are powered down. This ability to test the circuitry of the body was discovered by Dr. George Goodheart around 50 years ago. He found that through applied muscle testing, a trained physician can literally muscle test all the circuits of the body. It can determine quickly and accurately which parts of the nervous system, endocrine system, and acupuncture system are weak, disorganized, and powered down. Then muscle testing can determine the cause. Through a great deal of testing it became understood that multiple factors (allostatic stress) can accumulate to create disorganization to a level for circuits to trip. These factors include emotional stress, subluxations from injuries, poor lymphatic function, poor vascular flow, organ stress from low nutrition, food allergies, blocked detoxification pathways, and blocked cerebral spinal fluid due to poor cranial/sacral movement.

Applied kinesiology is akin to an electrician using meters to measure the electrical flow through a house. You wouldn't want an electrician to just guess which circuits are working and which are not. When it comes down to it, almost all physicians just guess and proceed to treat with toxic medications. Many doctors listen carefully to the patient's story, examine the body, do blood work, and then guess at what therapies may help.

Applied kinesiology takes away the guesswork. Through muscle testing, one can literally check which vertebra should be adjusted and in what direction, what nutrition should be increased, and which foods eliminated. Many even combine kinesiology with psychology to find the core emotions weakening a person.

Applied kinesiology remains one of the greatest human advancements in health, and I believe within 20 years all holistic physicians will be using it diagnostically. I believe Goodheart deserves the Nobel Prize for his discovery. The reasons so few have heard of him and so few physicians use applied kinesiology are twofold. First, muscle testing is an art along with a science, and becoming competent at muscle testing takes years of training.

Secondly, as with almost all natural cures, there is no large force of money that is being used to promote this to the masses. It is spreading by its own merit and word of mouth. The most common healing art using applied kinesiology is chiropractic, as it fits in perfectly as a measuring tool to determine which spinal vertebra are out and which adjustments are needed to restore function.

Thankfully recent developments in the world of computers and electronics have made it possible to use a biofeedback machine to "muscle" test the body efficiently and quickly.

I did not turn a corner with my health until I found a good kinesiologist. He guided me in correcting many of the structural twists in my spine still remaining from my car accident. He proceeded to identify that I had parasites, showed me that I was allergic to both dairy and gluten, and helped me implement many of the principles found in this book.

To the person suffering, finding a good applied kinesiologist or someone who is using a biofeedback

256

machines can be a lifesaver. The website listing applied kinesiologist physicians is the International College of Applied Kinesiology and their website is www.icakusa.com.

CHIROPRACTIC

The term chiropractic, for many, often evokes emotion. Many of us reject it while having very little understanding of what it is and how it works. We reject it because we had too many blue pills shoved down our throats. Chiropractic is the only way I've ever encountered of removing subluxations within the nervous system. It is evident that most people don't understand chiropractic by the mere fact that only 7% of people use it and even less understand it. Many adherents just know it makes them feel better. The purpose of chiropractic is simple—it seeks to increase the Universal Intelligence energy and nerve flow of the body, thus allowing the body to be more efficient at healing itself.

Spinal manipulation has been done for thousands of years in Asia, but the modern version and term chiropractic is relatively young. A man named D.D. Palmer discovered its principles one day in Iowa in the late 1800s. He met a man who had fallen off his horse years earlier and as a result had both neck pain and lost his hearing. Palmer made a manipulation in that man's neck, and as the story goes the man's hearing was immediately restored. The simple realization was born: Our nervous system controls everything and spinal manipulation is the way of increasing its function. Since that time, millions of people have been healed via spinal manipulation.

Numerous studies and data that show that chiropractic is beneficial for virtually every condition with no side effects. Most of the bad press from chiropractic has been engineered by Rockefeller Medicine and the American Medical Association (AMA). In fact, in the 1980s the chiropractic profession successfully sued the AMA for purposely trying to destroy the chiropractic profession for their own economic gain. Since the time of the Flexnor report, the AMA held that "unscientific practitioners" should be persecuted. In 1987 the AMA lost in court for violating the Sherman Act by engaging in unlawful conspiracy "to contain and eliminate the chiropractic profession."[117] This, however, has not stopped them from continuously putting out press in an effort to steer all patients away from chiropractic and down the prescription medication path.

Even if you increase all other aspects of health discussed so far in this book (mind, nutrition, digestion, breathing, movement, water, etc), the body will still not heal if its energy flow is disrupted. This necessitates that the patient work with a chiropractor, body worker, or acupuncturist. All professions work to accomplish the same objective. I happened to be trained in chiropractic and manipulation of the body and have found it to be an excellent method for balancing the body.

When seeking out a body worker, look for one that uses applied kinesiology muscle testing. Find one, listen to them, and follow their treatment plan. If the healer is competent you *will* get results. Results are the only thing that matter. If you don't get results within one month, seek out a different healer. You'll know when you find the right one! Depending on the severity of individual issues, it will take time to restore functionality. Some people are initially in more discomfort during the first week while the body is "turning back on." This is normal.

With chiropractic, many people require regular adjustments for one year before the nervous system and flow of energy can fully function. If permanent damage has occurred in the spine from arthritis, birth defects, injuries or other factors, then the patient will benefit from adjustments for life to maintain functionality. For the purposes of the 21 days of this program, get adjusted every day you are able. The constant input into your nervous system with the adjustments will dramatically increase the flow of energy through the body and assist the healing process.

23 - CBD OIL

ELEMENT—FIRE

REMOVE: Prescription medications
ADD IN: CBD Oil

"One of the first duties of the physician is to educate the masses not to take medicine."

—Sir William Osler

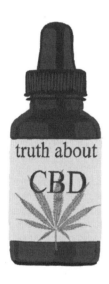

If you've done all the steps up to this point and are still plagued by symptoms of poor health (pain, infection, depression, cancer, etc) then cannabinoids, some of the ingredients of the cannabis plant, can often quite effectively replace other medications. If previously influenced by dogma or propaganda, you may want to reject this proposition because of the history of this plant. I too once looked at cannabis as a dangerous drug. Once I learned about the health benefits of cannabinoids, the history of the cannabis plant, and how to utilize it without the psychoactive side effects, I was forced to change my opinion.

Throughout history up until 90 years ago, cannabis was, as today, used widely. It was both consumed for recreation and prescribed as an effective medicinal plant. It's cousin, the hemp plant, is still used to make rope, paper, biofuel, and thousands of other products. Its broad uses were accepted in most quarters of society, including medicine. I've read accounts where doctors at the turn of the century would effectively prescribe meat and cannabis when they couldn't figure out what ailed a patient. Many of our forefathers grew it and used it. Thomas Jefferson wrote in his papers, "Some of my finest hours have been spent on my back veranda, smoking hemp, and observing as far as my eye can see."[118]

It was so widely used and grown with such ease that it is often referred to as weed. In many ways (health, environment, energy, farming, industrial uses) it is the perfect plant. Most open-minded people realize that nothing that shows up on Earth other than human greed is inherently bad, as all species co-evolved in an altruistic manner.

All this changed during the Rockefeller shift, as the destructive forces of human greed turned an evil eye towards cannabis, in an effort to destroy all competition in the 1930s. At this point in American history, Henry Ford was creating the first affordable car. To power his automobile, Henry Ford was experimenting with multiple forms of fuel including bio-fuels created from hemp. This, of course, directly threatened Rockefeller's gasoline sales. Since hemp also makes superior paper products, it was an enemy to the wood pulp industry and Andrew Hearst's paper mills. The therapeutic health benefits of cannabis threatened medicines emerging from pharmaceutical businesses. Through an unholy alliance, a campaign was created to destroy the competition that cannabis and hemp represented.

With the intention of destroying their competition, the alliance rolled out an anti-cannabis smear campaign. The term "marijuana," which was derived from the

Mexican slang term "marihuana," was purposely popularized by the Federal Bureau of Narcotics (which would later become the DEA) in order to invoke fear of the substance. The now hilariously campy "Reefer Madness" films and advertisements were widely distributed. Hurst's yellow journalism fanned the propaganda flame and exploited racist fears of minorities taking advantage of white women after getting them to smoke marijuana. Not unlike today, a good marketer or politician who does not have facts on his side will predictably use fear, prejudice, and ignorance to do their dirty work. Then, as now, these tactics greatly influenced an uninformed public.

The new prohibition law was a rather easy sell to a Congress that was snugly ensconced in the deep pockets of Rockefeller and Hearst. They purposely lumped hemp prohibition in with cannabis, and with it a major source of revenue for many American farmers went up in smoke. Hemp and cannabis were now officially removed as competition for Rockefeller's industrial empire. His lockdown of total control of the oil and pharmaceutical industries was set. Since that time, the Rockefeller family has profited greatly as hundreds of billions of pounds of petroleum and petroleum-based chemicals and pharmaceuticals have been distributed and used throughout the world. The Rockefeller family's influence on the world has enriched the family beyond countable assets, yet contributed to serious social decay throughout the entire hierarchy of classes and life. With this shift, we're witnessing skyrocketing rates of chronic disease, climate change, and a massive reduction in biodiversity of all animal life.

If you can't tell by now, I'm not a huge fan of Rockefeller. The greed that drove his life deserves denigration and is the origin of most of what is wrong with our world. I think his name shouldn't be spoken with admiration of his life and wealth and industrialism, but with anger and sadness right along with the most notorious criminals in history. His life should be rewritten for the truth that it was. Any monuments to him should be torn down or renamed, including the Rockefeller obelisk at his grave in Lake View Cemetery, overlooking and disgracing my home town of Cleveland, Ohio.

Making cannabis illegal has only contributed to the downward spiral of American life by placing millions of people in jail for its growth and use, destabilizing most especially the African American community. I can only begin to speculate how much taxpayer money has been spent and how many lives have been lost on law enforcement, prisons, loss of revenue to the farmers, industry, and healthcare by this Rockefeller shift. Yet through it all, the fact remains that cannabis and hemp plants are highly beneficial, and as far as I know has never killed even a single person. All the studies of the potential positive benefits of cannabis and hemp come from other countries, while the United States is notably silent on the subject. Here follows the truth about cannabis.

POSITIVE EFFECTS OF CANNABIS

The short history of how much effort has been exercised to prevent the average American's access to cannabis should inspire the reader of its power. Many people are astounded to hear that cannabis produces a substance identical to the human body that is required for human health. These compounds are called the Endogenous Cannabinoids or Endocannabinoids. In the mid-1990s, Dr. Ralph Mechaoulam, a renowned Israeli researcher and professor of medicinal chemistry at Hebrew University in Jerusalem, made an exciting discovery that would forever change how we look at our biological relationship to the cannabis plant. Mechaoulam discovered a subtle system within the body that has a balancing effect on every other system. He called it the Endocannabinoid (EC) System and found receptors present on the cells of all mammals on earth.

When Mechaoulam discovered the Endocannabinoid system, he stated "There is barely a biological, physiological system in our bodies in which the endocannabinoids do not participate." He went on to say that he believes the cannabinoids are essential nutrients that the body needs to overcome chronic stress and balance the body's systems. Dr. Ethan Russo, a cannabinoid researcher, agrees and has stated that many diseases are created by a deficiency within the Endocannabinoid system now being called, "Clinical Endocannabinoid Deficiency Syndrome."

The Endocannabinoid system has been found to affect the release of neurotransmitters, immune function, the periphery nervous system, and the inflammatory system. So far at least 85 different cannabinoids in plants have been found to affect our cellular response. The receptors for these cannabinoids are found in the highest concentration in the brain, peripheral nervous system, immune system, and spleen. Our bodies are only able to produce small amounts cannabinoids (CBDs), which seems insufficient to handle modern-day stress for many people. Because of this, people with conditions like anxiety, depression, neurological diseases, chronic pain and inflammation, arthritis, cardiovascular disease, cancer, and PTSD have found a great deal of relief from cannabis.

Research is identifying that the cannabinoid receptors on our cells actually have a higher affinity to plant cannabinoids than from the cannabinoids the body produces. When the body comes in contact with therapeutic doses of CBDs, it triggers a series of cellular responses including apoptosis (preprogrammed cell death) to sick cells by stopping cells from dividing. Apoptosis comes from the Greek term which translates to "the falling away of leaves." Many find, when beginning to take CBDs, that they feel groggy and tired as the body selectively clears out the sick cells.

Cannabinoids have been shown extremely effective in healing cancer via inhibition of the GPR55 signaling system. The GPR55 system is mostly found inside the brain and is associated with blood pressure regulation, modulating bone density, and preventing the proliferation of cancer.[119] Microbiologist Dr. Christine Sanchez of Compultenese University of Madrid was one of the first to discover the anti-cancer effects of cannabinoids. She states in a video interview on a web-based video channel called *Cannabis Planet:* "We now know that the Endocannabinoid system regulates a lot of biological functions such as appetite, food intake, motor function, reproduction, and many others, and that is why the plant has such wide therapeutic potential." She has gone on to state, "One of the advantages of cannabinoid-based medicines would be that they target specifically tumor cells. They don't have any toxic effect on normal, non-tumor cells. This is an advantage with respect to standard chemotherapy that targets basically everything." The CBD system programs diseased tumor cells to "autophagy" and consume themselves, which stimulates the regeneration of healthy new cells. A search on *Pubmed*, the national open-access system for reporting the results of studies, shows roughly 500 articles relating to cannabis and cancer.

RATIO OF CBDs and THC

While the research is still in its infancy, the people I've spoken with, the books I've read, the videos I've watched, and the patients I've talked to about cannabis, it seems that the most effective way to consume cannabinoids is in a balanced ratio THC and CBDs. THC, or tetrahydrocannabinol, is the cannabinoid in cannabis responsible for the euphoric high. Plants can be bred to naturally contain a balanced ratio of both and when it does it creates what's called an "entourage effect." This entourage effect is much more effective than consuming THC or CBD by themselves. The levels of CBD and THC in plants can range from 5% to 15% and the goal is to find a balanced ratio. Many cannabis plants today have been bred to be high only in THC as many people are unaware of the health befits of non-psychoactive CBD.

If your primary complaints are seizures, depression, anxiety, or spasms, the dose of CBD should be higher than the THC. If you are treating cancer, neurological diseases, PTSD and most other conditions the ratio of CBD/THC should be closer to 1:1.

BUT I DON'T WANT TO GET HIGH

Neither do I, and proper supplementation doesn't get you high. Here's why: THC-A is what naturally comes from a plant. Only once heat is applied to the carboxylic acids (the last -A) from the carbon chain are the -A acids removed. In an unheated form there is no bio-activation, which is what is responsible for the high. THC is widely know as the cannabinoid that gets you high. People smoke, cook, or vaporize the THC-A to activate it through heat to get the psychological effects of THC. THC-A, the unheated compound, is highly effective at a biological level and doesn't get the user high. Also, when THC is accompanied by CBD, there is far less likelihood of getting high. If you don't want to get high, don't heat the compounds or just consume straight CBD oil. CBD doesn't get you high at all. Using a high CBD, unheated compound should not result in a "buzz". I don't think it's a good idea to heat the compound or use high THC and get high. Doing so changes the compound and I find getting "stoned" often becomes a crutch to patients that stops them from taking real action in their life. Without the high, you can objectively determine if it's helping or not.

THE BEST METHOD FOR CONSUMING CANNABIS

The best way to get the widest range of benefits from cannabis is through a cold pressed extraction method. This preserves all the health compounds and contributes to the beneficial "entourage effect." People either soak the plants in alcohol or oil, such as fractionated coconut oil or olive oil. This extraction can carry as many as 400 different CBD's, and trace compounds that are beneficial to health.

HOW MUCH SHOULD I TAKE

When the plant is cold extracted, the final product will have a varying amount of CBD. A therapeutic dose can very greatly. It's generally accepted to take between 2.5-25mg daily.

Each dose will last for approximately six hours in the system so the best protocol is to dose every six hours. Feel free to play with the dose as many people normalize at a much smaller or larger dose.

BEWARE OF FAKE PRODUCTS

CBD oil works better if it's from a real cannabis plant and not industrial hemp. Most of what's being sold in the market is industrial hemp. Cannabis is still illegal in many states so many have no choice but to use CBD from hemp. There is strong scientific evidence that industrial hemp CBD does not carry nearly the benefit that a natural cannabis plant carries. Most notable is the lack of the "entourage effect" that seems to carry the CBD to the cell receptors where it can activate cellular response. As with all compounds, quality matters. Finding the real thing can be a challenge if you live in a state where cannabis is still illegal. Cannabis, like all substances, can be toxic if grown in bad soil and treated with artificial fertilizers and chemicals. It's very important to know your source.

LEGALITY

No substance created by nature is innately bad. Some are poisonous and can kill you, while others have the ability to stimulate great healing. For the last 100 years, those in power have created a profit-driven war on some drugs, some of the time. When they can't figure out how to make money on a drug, plant, or commodity, or it competes with other forms of revenue, it's made illegal, subjugated, or made the target of a viscous smear campaign. It's clearly a system that operates with a series of double standards.

Cannabis and its receptors are clearly a natural ingredient in the fabric of human health. I find it no coincidence that since the time it has been made illegal, disease rates have soared. What could be a more obvious example of our society's separation from health than how we approach the cannabis plant?

Cannabis is currently legal in 25 states for medical purposes. If cannabis is still illegal in your state and you feel the need to try it, make arrangements to find it or go to a state where it is legal to consume. If you are unable to do this, start with the cannabinoids found in hemp.

HEALTH SIDE EFFECTS

The U.S. government states that there are no signs of toxicity or serious side effects from consuming cannabis. This is clearly evident from the fact that there has never been a recorded death from consuming cannabis. If using activated THC, the user should not operate a vehicle as it can affect neurological response times. I recommend avoid activating the THC by consuming the cold-pressed compound.

WHY THIS IS MENTIONED LAST

The reason I've mentioned cannabis last is that cannabis is nature's medication. Medication should always be used as a last resort after diet and lifestyle changes have been made. The use of medicine without changes in diet and lifestyle will not provide lasting healing. If medicine must be used, I would far rather have patients using a natural compound with a myriad of health benefits than a destructive man-made pharmaceutical. Please allow your own conscience and personal needs dictate your use of this plant and, like all medicines, use it respectfully and prudently.

24 - THE CONCLUSION

If you finished this book and choose to apply the healing techniques within, then you're one of those who is looking for a better life. You may be plagued with illness or pain, or just know that there is a better way to live. You may have realized that a system has been forced on us by a society that is living out of balance with nature and motivated by greed. You may have been mistreated, abused, lied to, or taught to believe that we somehow don't deserve to lead a life of rich happiness and health. Seeing the chains is the most painful part: it is the awakening. After you see the chains, forgive those who put them on you and then take them off.

You are on the journey of the Whole Body Health Warrior. It takes many twists and turns through life. Perhaps you'll wonder at times on this path if you can bear it. You may be in a rough patch right now. Someday you will look back on your journey and realize that you had to go through the rough patches. I had to go through them, you have to go through them, as everyone who learns anything does. We needed to see the darkness so that we can understand the light. We needed to know pain and sickness so we can understand and appreciate health. We had to go through hate so we can feel and realize love.

If going through this journey of pain brings you to a place of realizing love for yourself, this beautiful planet, and God, then it was and is completely worth it.

OK, it's time for your rocket ship of new health to take off. A bit more advice before I go!

Open your mind to new possibilities of healing and life. Try to drop all preconceived paradigms and beliefs that got you sick. Instead, believe and know that you are healed. Completely healed. Speak words of power over your life. You have the choice to create your life; choose the path less traveled by. Choose to be a warrior of truth. Run from zombies—zombie medicine, toxic zombie people, zombie food, zombie water and zombie air. Try to conserve your energy from these zombies, as they are like openings in a reservoir that will quickly waste your vital waters.

Instead, spend as much of your life as you are able in nature. Take off your shoes and walk through the forests. Take off your clothes and swim in the ocean. Turn off the TV and lay out under the stars and stare into the cosmos. Have fun and laugh as often as you are able. Try to always be grateful. After all, what's your other choice?

Treat your body as a temple and work to constantly increase its cellular energy. Give it good organic food raised in a morally conscious and sustainable manner. Live in a high vibration space with clean air, alive water, and lots of sunshine. Create that space.

Move every day as much as you can in ways that challenge you and bring you joy. Never stop breathing! When that's not enough, find a healer whose talent works for you. Allow that person to remove your blockages and walk you through the process of healing.

Dale Carnegie said, "Most of the important things in the world have been accomplished by people who have kept on trying when there seemed to be no hope at all." So must importantly I say this to you: Never stop pushing, never give up hope!

Once you heal, work to help lift others. I wish you lots of love, hope, and Whole Body Health. God Bless.
-Dr. Tim Weeks

APPENDIX A: PHASE I FOODS

NO LIMIT:
Protein:
Meat
Fish
Fowl
Eggs
Fats (See below for a list)
Vegetables that have less that 9% carbohydrate in them. (See below for a list)
Apple cider vinegar
Raw nuts (no more than one cup per day and not peanuts)
Water (spring or filtered - preferably structured)
Non Caffeine Teas
Bone Broth
Fermented Vegetables and Drinks

AVOID COMPLETELY:
Grains
Fruit
Alcohol
Soybean Oil
Canola Oil
Milk

UNLIMITED VEGETABLES:
3% or less carbohydrate

Asparagus

Bamboo Shoots

Bean Sprouts

Beet Greens

Bok Choy Greens

Broccoli

Cabbages

Celery

Chards

Miracle Noodles ?

Collard Greens

Chestnuts

Brussel Sprouts

Turnips

Onion

Mushrooms

7-9% Carbohydrate

Mustard Greens

Parsley

Radishes

Salad Greens

Spinach

Yellow Squash

Kimchi

6% or less

Bell Peppers

Chives

Eggplant

Green Beans

Okra

Olives

Pickles

Pimento

Rhubarb

Tomatoes

Water

Cucumber

Garlic

Kale

Lettuces

Acorn Squash

Artichokes

Avocado

Beets

Carrots

UNLIMITED FATS:
Butter
Ghee
Coconut Oil
Lard/Bacon Grease/Tallow/Duck Fat
Olive Oil ✓
Sesame Seed Oil
Walnut Oil

APPENDIX B: WEEK OF MEALS (examples)

Day 1
Breakfast:
2 Eggs over easy cooked in butter/coconut oil
2 pieces uncured bacon

Lunch:
1 glass fresh juiced vegetables

Dinner:
Bun-free grass-fed burger with cooked mushrooms, onions.
Sautéed mixed veggies cooked in coconut oil

Day 2
Breakfast:
Nuclear fusion coffee/atomic tea (see appendix C)

Lunch:
Mixed green salad topped with chicken and veggies.
Salad dressing of apple cider vinegar and organic olive oil.

Dinner:
Low carb marinara sauce with ground beef or meatballs on top of spaghetti squash

Day 3
Breakfast:
2 Egg muffins (recipe provided)
1 glass vegetable juice

Lunch:
Guacamole and cut up carrots

Dinner:
Grass-fed steak topped with butter. Season with pepper and Himalayan salt.
Loaded cauliflower mash (recipe provided)

Day 4
Breakfast:
Egg omelette with cooked mushrooms, onions, red peppers and spinach

Lunch:
Chicken patty topped with red peppers and fried egg

Dinner:
Root vegetables roasted in coconut oil. Fresh vegetable juice.

Day 5
Breakfast:
Keto pancakes topped with butter (recipe provided)

Lunch:
BLT in lettuce wrap. Fresh vegetable juice

Dinner:
Baked chicken breast topped with uncured pepperoni and mozzarella cheese.
Side of broccoli sautéed in coconut oil

Day 6
Breakfast:
Eggs with bacon. Fresh Vegetable juice.

Lunch:
Zucchini noodles topped with butter with grilled chicken

Dinner:
Cheese crust pizza (recipe provided)

Day 7
Breakfast:
Atomic tea

Lunch:

Green smoothie with cucumber, carrots, kale, beets, half lemon. Vegetable salad.

Dinner:

Roasted Chicken thighs and vegetables cooked in olive oil. (Beetroot, carrot, onion, Brussels sprouts, sweet potatoes)

Snacks:

Sliced carrots with guacamole

Nuts/seeds limited to ¼ cup per day

String cheese

Celery with nut butter on top

Uncured pepperoni

Beef sticks (read ingredients — no sugar, MSG, nitrites or artificial flavors)

Fermented veggies

APPENDIX C: RECIPES

LIQUID DRINKS

Atomic Tea:

1-2 TBSP coconut oil
1-2 TBSP grass-fed butter
2 TBSP gelatin/collagen
1 scoop vanilla bone broth protein powder from Ancient Nutrition.
14 oz hot tea (any flavor) decaf or regular
Charged Fulvic and Humic Minerals—1 dropper full
Optional: Cacao butter, cacao powder, unsweetened coconut milk, CBD oil
Mix well in blender

Nuclear Fusion Coffee:

1-2 TBSP coconut oil
1-2 TBSP grass fed butter
1 TBSP gelatin/collagen
14 oz hot coffee
Charged Fulvic and Humic Minerals—1 dropper full
Optional: Cacao butter, cacao powder, unsweetened coconut milk, CBD oil
Mix well in blender.

These cups of coffee or tea are jam packed with minerals, collagen, and fat! YUMMO! The fat, caffeine, minerals, and CBD combine in a way that makes your brain explode with energy. It is the ultimate energy drink and healing beverage.

Bone Broth

- 4-5 pounds of bones, preferably marrow and knuckle bones.

- if using beef bones, add in a calf foot cut into pieces (optional)

- if using chicken broth, add in chicken heads and feet (optional)

- 4 quarts of filtered water, or as much as needed to just cover the bones

- 1/2 cup apple cider vinegar

- 2 onions chopped

- 6 carrots chopped

- 6 stalks of celery chopped

- 1 sprig of fresh thyme tied together

- 1 bunch of parsley

- Place bones in a large pot with water and vinegar and allow to sit for 1 hours. The water should just cover the bones—too much and it won't gel. Bring to a boil and then reduce heat to a low simmer. The water should just be rolling but not boiling. A scum will rise to the surface. This is normal. Remove it with a slotted spoon. Allow it to simmer for 24-48 hours.

- Remove the bones. Allow the broth to cool outside if it's winter or in the refrigerator to allow the fat on the top to harden. Once congealed, remove it and save for cooking or discard. Strain broth to remove sediment and then enjoy.

Beet Kavass

2 large beets
1/4 cup fermented whey, juice from sauerkraut, kombucha or kvass to get it started
1 tablespoon sea salt (non iodized)
1/2 gallon pitcher or jar
filtered water

Wash beets, cut them into 1/2 inch cubes and place in a glass jar. Add in a few ounces of liquid fermented starter and salt. Fill with filtered water and cover with a towel so it can breathe. In one to two days it will be finished, depending on temperature. Then pour out liquid and put in the refrigerator. Beets can be used twice. So after you pour out the water, fill it up with water and salt again and leave it for another two days.

If you leave it out too long it will get something that looks like mold on top. Simply scrape this off, add a little more salt and move liquid to refrigerator.

BREAKFAST

Egg Muffins

6 eggs, beaten
salt/pepper to taste
1-2 TBSP heavy whipping cream
½ cup shredded cheddar cheese
Chopped veggies (peppers, onions, mushrooms, etc.)
Sausage patty

Line a muffin tin with sausage patty to make a "cup." Cook at 350 degrees for 10-15 minutes. In the meantime, beat together egg, cream, salt/pepper, veggies and cheese.

When sausage is done, pour the egg mixture into muffin tins on top of the sausage. Cook for 30 minutes or until the egg has set. Other options: you can use chopped, cooked, uncured bacon added to egg mixture.

Sausage Breakfast Casserole

1 lb pork sausage
2 cups diced zucchini
2 cups green cabbage, shredded
½ diced onion
3 large eggs
½ cup avocado mayonnaise
2 tsp yellow mustard
1 tsp ground sage
1 ½ cups cheddar cheese, shredded (optional)
cayenne pepper to taste

Preheat oven to 375 degrees and grease casserole pan. Brown sausage in large skillet over medium heat until almost cooked through. Add cabbage, zucchini and onion, cooking until vegetables are tender and sausage fully cooked. Remove from heat and spoon into prepared casserole dish, then set aside. In a mixing bowl, whisk eggs, mayonnaise, mustard, sage, and pepper until smooth. Add a cup of grated cheese to egg mixture and stir. Pour this mixture over the sausage and vegetables in the casserole dish. Top casserole with remaining ½ cup cheese (optional). Place casserole in preheated oven and bake 30 minutes, or until bubbling around the edges and cheese is melted. Remove from oven and serve immediately.

Keto Pancakes

4 oz cream cheese
4 eggs
Cinnamon
Vanilla (or few drops of vanilla stevia)

Blend ingredients well. Pour thin mixture in coconut oil to make what will look like a crepe. Keep it thin and small as it will continue to spread. Flip after a few minutes like you would a pancake until both sides are golden brown.

Note: you can do without the cinnamon and vanilla, adding any spice to mimic tortilla shell or wrap.

Almond Flour Pancakes

1 ½ cups almond flour
3 eggs
1 cup of water or unsweetened coconut milk
cinnamon, nutmeg to taste

Mix all ingredients in a bowl using a hand blender or immersion blender until batter is pourable. Cook all pancakes on griddle or large pan in butter or coconut oil for approximately 2-3 min per side or until bubbles form.

Country Gravy

4 oz sausage
2 TBSP butter
1 cup heavy cream
salt and pepper to taste

Add sausage to pan and let brown. Remove when fully cooked. Add 2 TBSP butter to the pan and let it melt. Then, add heavy cream to the pan, stirring as it bubbles. Add sausage back into the pan and stir together. Serve over almond flour muffins if so desired.

Almond Flour Muffins

2 ½ cups almond flour
2 TBSP coconut flour
1 TBSP stevia or xylitol
1 tsp salt
2 tsp baking powder
½ cup mozzarella
10 egg whites

Beat 10 egg whites until frothy then add the other ingredients until well mixed. Cut in six TBSP cold butter until well mixed. Portion out into 12 muffin tins. Bake at 400 degrees for 10-12 minutes or until golden brown.

MEAL IDEAS

Hot Spinach Salad

1 large box of Spinach - or any other green — kale, chard, etc.
4 TBSP apple cider vinegar
2 small beets
4 carrots
1 large or 2 small onions
8 cups cut up mushrooms
4 cloves garlic
Salt to taste
6 TBSP coconut oil

Cut up onions, mushrooms and garlic. Shred beets and carrots. Put coconut oil in frying pan and cook onions until they begin to caramelize. When they are beginning to brown, add in garlic, mushrooms, carrots and beets. After everything is cooked, add in spinach. Continue to cook until greens are soft and warm. Add in apple cider vinegar and salt to taste.

Green Tuna Salad

Greens—spinach or romaine
Red onions
Olives
Carrot
Canned line-caught tuna
Olive oil
Apple cider vinegar
Any other vegetable
Combine all ingredients and enjoy!

Root Vegetables

Brussels sprouts
Fennel
Carrots
Garlic
Onions
Cauliflower
Olive oil or coconut oil
Green Beans
Salt

Chicken Legs or Thighs (optional)

Cut up vegetables and place them on a roasting pan. Thoroughly coat everything with oil. Add salt to taste.

Add chicken legs or thighs if you like. Roast at 400 degrees for 1 hour or until everything is cooked, soft and slightly browned.

Salmon and Green Beans

Wild caught salmon
Green beans
Salt
Lemon pepper
Olive oil
Butter

Coat salmon in olive oil. Sprinkle with salt and lemon pepper. Heat more olive oil in a pan and then place salmon in pan. Cook for approximately five minutes on each side. This will very depending on thickness of salmon and heat of pan.

Steam greened beans for 10 minutes. Add salt and butter to taste.

Sweet Potato French Fries

Sweet potatoes
Olive Oil
Salt
Sugar-free ketchup

Cut up sweet potatoes in wedges. Place on a baking sheet and cover both sides with olive oil. Salt to taste. Roast vegetables at 350 degrees for 45 minutes to an hour depending on thickness of vegetables.

Crock Pot Chicken

Whole pastured organic chicken
Onions
Mushroom
Fennel
Garlic
Carrots
Salt

Place entire chicken in a crock pot. Surround with all the vegetables. Turn crock pot on low for eight hours or high for four hours.

Chicken Divan Casserole

16 oz broccoli florets
4 cooked chicken breasts
3 cups avocado mayonnaise
2 TBSP curry powder
Juice form 2 lemons
1 cup grated Parmesan
cheese (optional)
¼ cup melted butter

Preheat oven to 350 degrees. Place broccoli florets in bottom of casserole pan. Cover broccoli with chicken. Mix together mayonnaise, curry powder, and lemon juice. Spread mayonnaise mixture over chicken. Sprinkle parmesan evenly over chicken. Pour melted butter over parmesan and bake for 45 minutes.

Unstuffed Cabbage Rolls

1 ½ - 2 lbs grass-fed ground beef
1 small cabbage, chopped

1 TBSP butter
30 oz diced tomatoes
1 large onion, chopped
8 oz tomato sauce
1 clove garlic, chopped
1 tsp salt
1 tsp pepper

In large skillet heat butter, ground meat, onion and cook until meat cooked and onion tender. Add garlic. Add chopped cabbage, tomatoes, tomato sauce, salt, and pepper. Bring to a boil, reduce heat and simmer for 20-30 min.

APPENDIX D: ALLERGY ELIMINATION

First you must determine if you have a food sensitivity and there are four self methods you can use to determine what foods your sensitive to.

Muscle Test - Having a trained kinesiologist muscle test you will quickly and accurately determine which foods your body is sensitive to. This is most accurate test available. Many people, with a little training, can learn to muscle test.

Cocoa Pulse Test - Take your pulse before you eat a suspicious food and again 15 and 30 minutes after eating. If your sensitive, your pulse rate is going to go up as the adrenals and immune system respond. The higher the rise the more sensitive you are.

How you feel test. This is just what it sounds like. After you finish the 21 days of phase 1 of the Whole Body Health formula, start slowly bringing back potentially allergic foods (dairy, grains, etc.). Keep a journal of how you feel. If any of your health complaints come back or you notice a response look back at what you ate. Through this method you can figure out what foods your body is still reacting to.

Sway Test - You have to be somewhat sensitive to your own energy to perform this, but for many this is an invaluable test. The way you perform this is to stand with your feet together (preferably without shoes on). Put the substance or food in your hand and put it against your chest. Ask yourself the question, "Am I sensitive to this food?" and then let your body be either pulled forward or fall backwards. If you feel you body

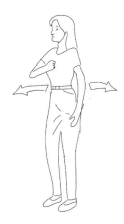

being pulled forward you are not sensitive, if you being pulled backward, there is strong likelihood of a sensitivity.

Natural Allergy Elimination Technique

Once you determine what foods your sensitive to you can "reset" these allergies.

This is the process:

1. Hold the food and get someone to rub the acupuncture points for 30 seconds each in the order listed:

2. Tap up and down the back for 5 minutes while breathing deeply in and out.

3. Continue to hold the substance for 15 minutes while laying quietly with the allergen in your hand on your chest.

4. Avoid the food or substance for 25 hours to allow your immune system to reset.

5. Recheck the sensitivity. Stronger sensitivities can often take multiple resets before your body forgets the food sensitivity.

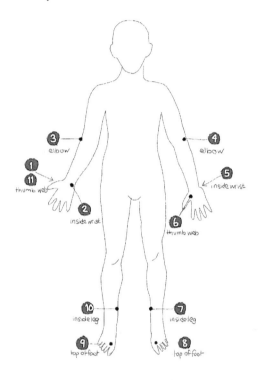

APPENDIX E: LIVER FLUSH INSTRUCTIONS

FOR ONE WEEK BEFORE FLUSH STARTS:

Take 9 Malic Acid tablets (available on Amazon) to help thin the bile.

1) Take 9 Liver Drainage per day (available on Whole Body Health website)

2) Avoid meat and fat

ON DAY OF FLUSH:

1) On day of flush eat no fat whatsoever. Food could consist of fresh squeezed juice, a sweet potato, and carrots

2) After lunch, place 4 tablespoons of Epsom salt (magnesium sulfate) dissolved in 3 cups of warm mineral water. Once dissolved, put it in the fridge.

3) Four hours after lunch, take a 1-quart coffee enema with one-fourth (1/4) cup of Epsom salt dissolved in it. This should be retained for 15 minutes and expelled. (see appendix F)

4) Five hours after lunch (5 p.m.) drink one cup of your prepared Epsom salt water. (The taste is not nice, but drink it anyway. It can be followed by a little citrus juice if needed.)

5) Eight hours after lunch (8 p.m.), drink another cup of Epsom salt water.

6) At bedtime, take one-half (1/2) cup of unrefined olive oil mixed with 1/2 cup fresh-squeezed orange, grapefruit,

or lemon juice. Put in a jar and shake it to mix the juice and oil together (this will make it much easier to drink). Drink the combination.

7) Immediately upon drinking the oil, go to bed and lie on the right side with the right knee pulled up toward the chest for 30 minutes. This encourages the oil to drain from the stomach, helping contents of the gall bladder and liver to move into the small intestine.

8) If you feel quite ill during the night, take another strong coffee enema with one-fourth (1/4) cup of Epsom salt dissolved in it.

9) If there is a strong feeling of nausea the following morning, try to remain in bed until it subsides. Do not force vomiting.

NEXT DAY:

1) Upon rising drink, consume the last cup of Epsom salt water.

2) Then take another strong coffee enema.

Expect to have diarrhea until about 2 p.m. the next day. Try to plan ahead so you don't have to leave the house. In your stool, look for floating green stones. These are from the gall bladder. They are green because bile is green and float because they are full of cholesterol and fat. If you don't get stones out, it doesn't mean that you don't have them. Often it can take doing a liver flush several times before the liver is able to release. The liver flush should be repeated monthly until health is restored and you are no longer releasing stones. Once health is restored, it should be performed twice per year.

APPENDIX F: COFFEE ENEMA INSTRUCTIONS

PREPARE THE COFFEE

1) The coffee must be organic, regular coffee. Make it as strong as possible.

The traditional drip coffee is fine. Don't use your Keurig. In fact, drop this off at the Salvation Army!

2) The water should be RO, filtered or distilled water. If you don't have access to this, get it right now. This is true of your drinking and bathing water as well.

3) The coffee enema should consist of 1 quart of coffee, held for 15 minutes, as this is how long it takes to get all the blood of the body to flow through the liver.

HOW TO TAKE THE COFFEE ENEMA

1) Attempt a normal bowel movement before starting the enema. The enema is much more effective if the colon has been emptied. If unable to do this, do a water enema first to get the stool out, then start the coffee enema.

2) Again, use RO, filtered or distilled water.

3) When it is completed, the coffee retention enema may be performed.

4) Begin the 1 quart of coffee in your enema bag or bucket.

5) Next, allow the coffee to flow to the end of the colon tube, thus eliminating any air in the tube.

6) The colon tube should be lubricated with natural oil, butter, or other lubricant that doesn't contain chemicals.

7) Lie on the left side until the coffee is completely retained.

8) After the coffee enema is completed, remove the tip from inside you. Lie on your left side for another 7-10 minutes, then lie on your back for 7-10 minutes.

9) After the enema is retained for 15 minutes or longer, you may release it.

REFERENCES

1 Summary Health Statistics for U.S. Adults: National Health Interview Survey, 2012, table 35[PDF – 1.3 MB] www.cdc.gov/nchs/data/series/sr_10/sr10_260.pdf

2 https://seer.cancer.gov/statfacts/html/all.html

3 https://www.cdc.gov/nchs/data/databriefs/db50.htm

4 https://www.cdc.gov/media/pressrel/2010/r101022.html

5 https://www.cancer.gov/types/childhood-cancers/child-adolescent-cancers-fact-sheet

6 http://www.motherearthnews.com/natural-health/male-fertility-crisis-zmaz83sozraw

7 Weitz, Martin, "Health Shock"

8 http://data.worldbank.org/indicator/SP.DYN.IMRT.IN?year_high_desc=false

9 http://www.who.int/whr/2000/en/

10 Ullman, Dana. "How Scientific is Modern Medicine, Really?" Pathways to Family Wellness, Issue #27. 2010

11 Duff, 2010. The New York Times.

12 https://en.m.wikipedia.org/wiki/Hippocrates

13 Muscles are weakened with just enough stress to gain strength in the long run.

14 The Global 2000 Report to the President, Volumes I and II, Blue Angel, Inc. July 1981

15 Weinhold B. Epigenetics: The Science of Change. *Environmental Health Perspectives*. 2006;114(3):A160-A167.

[16] To fully understand this concept of frequency and harmonic resonance, I highly recommend you read the book, "Power vs. Force" by Dr. David Hawkins.

17 http://ethics.harvard.edu/blog/new-prescription-drugs-major-health-risk-few-offsetting-advantages

[18] http://www.naturalnews.com/ 037226_drug_prescriptions_medical_news_pills.html#ixzz2Vl DeYjfo

19 Victor Luckerson, Time Magazine, Dec 17, 2015, Everything to Know About the Arrested Drug Price-Hiking CEO, website: http://time.com/4153512/martin-shkreli-pharmaceuticals-arrested-turing-daraprim/

20 http://www.webdc.com/pdfs/deathbymedicine.pdf

[21] 2006, Nutrition Institute of America; Independent Review. https://draxe.com/conventional-medicine-is-the-leading-cause-of-death/

[22] Soc Sci Med. 2008 Dec;67(11):1784-8. doi: 10.1016/ j.socscimed.2008.09.044. Epub 2008 Oct 10.

23 Doctors' strikes and mortality: A review. Solveig Argeseanu Cunningham, Kristina Mitchell, K.M. Venkat Narayan, Salim Yusuf. Social Science & Medicine 67 (2008) 1784-1788

24 *BMJ* 2012;345:e7191

25 http://www.wsj.com/articles/SB123552190314864789

26 http://www.bloomberg.com/bw/stories/2005-07-17/is-heart-surgery-worth-it

27 Mozzafarian D, Benjamin EJ, Go AS, et al. Heart Disease and Stroke Statistics-2015 Update: a report from the American Heart Association. Circulation. 2015;e29-322.

28 "$29 Billion Reasons to Lie About Cholesterol" Smith, Justin

29 http://www.webmd.com/healthy-aging/features/heart-disease-medical-costs

30 http://www.collective-evolution.com/2015/05/16/editor-in-chief-of-worlds-best-known-medical-journal-half-of-all-the-literature-is-false/

31 http://www.pbs.org/wgbh/pages/frontline/shows/other/interviews/angell.html

32 https://doi.org/10.1371/journal.pmed.0020124

33 "Rockefeller and His Medicine Men" Brown, E. Richard

34 http://www.goodreads.com/quotes/859052-i-will-never-attend-an-anti-war-rally-if-you-have

35 Chernow R. *Titan: The Life of John D Rockefeller Sr* (New York: Vintage Books, 2004), pp 471–2.

36 Ward O. Griffen, Jr, MD, PhD. "Jacob; The Other Flexner", *Annals of Surgery*, 2004 June; 239(6): 808–817, hosted at National Library of Medicine, NIH, accessed 23 October 2013

37 Heather I. *Rockefeller was big, and his doctor was Biggar (March 2011)*. Website :http://www.brantfordexpositor.ca/2011/03/05/rockefeller-was-big-and-his-doctor-was-biggar

38 Bonner, Thomas Neville (February 1998). "Searching for Abraham Flexner". *Academic Medicine*.

39 Abraham Flexner: An Autobiography, New York: Simon and Schuster, 1960

40 Beck AH (2004). "The Flexner Report and the standardization of American medical education". *JAMA*. **291** (17): 2139–2140. doi:10.1001/jama.291.17.2139. PMID 15126445.

41 http://www.ncbi.nlm.nih.gov/pmc/articles/PMC2967338/

42 http://www.nytimes.com/books/98/05/17/specials/rockefeller-gifts.html

43 http://www.huffingtonpost.com/dana-ullman/how-the-ama-got-rich-powe_b_6103720.html

44 Starr, P. The Social Transformation of American Medicine. New York: Basic Books, 1982

45 Fishbein, M. Morris Fishbein, MD: An Autobiography. New York: Doubleday, 1969

46 Bonner, Thomas Neville (February 1998). "Searching for Abraham Flexner". *Academic Medicine*. **73** (2): 160–166.

47 Duffy TP. The Flexner Report — 100 Years Later. *The Yale Journal of Biology and Medicine*. 2011;84(3):269-276.

48 Hanninen, O.; Farago, M.; Monos, E. (September–October 1983), "Ignaz Philipp Semmelweis, the prophet of bacteriology", *Infection Control*, 4 (5): 367–370

49 AARP. Beyond 50.2003: A Report to the Nation on Independent Living and Disability, 2003, <http://www.aarp.org/research/health/disabilities/aresearch-import-753.html> (11 Jan 2005).

50 U.S. Census Bureau, news release, May 6, 2014

51 Czarnikow, F O Licht, ISO, Board of Trade Journal; http://www.czarnikow.com/news/01-05-14/inconvenient-truth-about-sugar-consumption-it-s-not-what-you-think

52 "Harvey Wiley Explains Resignation" (PDF). The Daily Princetonian. Associated Press. March 16, 1912. p. 1. Arcived from the original on March 2009.

53 "Farm Subsidies Over Time". *The Washington Post*. 2 July 2006. Retrieved 12 April 2012
Stephen Vogel. "Farm Income and Costs: Farms Receiving Government Payments". Ers.usda.gov. Retrieved 12 April 2012

54 Andrew Cassel (6 May 2002). "Why U.S. Farm Subsidies Are Bad for the World". Philadelphia Inquirer. Archived from the original on 9 June 2007. Retrieved 20 July 2007.

55 "EWG Farm Subsidy Database". Farm.ewg.org. 29 November 2004. Retrieved 12 April 2012.

56 "EWG Farm Subsidy Database". Farm.ewg.org.

57 2005, Congressional Office Budget Report

58 http://www.pcrm.org

59 Philip Bump. "Lobbyist spent $173.5 million trying to shape the 2008 farm bill" www.grist.org. July 19, 2012

60 https://www.statista.com/statistics/257364/top-lobbying-industries-in-the-us/

61 Lillbert K etal. American J. Of Epidemioligy, 2003;157(5:415-23. Benninx Be, et al.
Journal of National Cancer Institute. 1998; 90(24):1999-92. Price.

62 Wampold BE, Minami T, Tierney SC, Baskin TW, Bhati KS; Minami; Tierney; Baskin; Bhati (2005). "The placebo is powerful: estimating placebo effects in medicine and psychotherapy from randomized clinical trials". *J Clin Psychol*. **61** (7): 835–54. doi:10.1002/jclp.20129. PMID 15827993.

63 "Do You Know What Your Patients Eat?" Monograph, E. Cheraskin, W. Ringsdorf, Dept. Oral Med., U. Alabama (1976).

64 https://www.merriam-webster.com/dictionary/poison

65 http://www.doctorofthefuture.org/archives/Y2006/august/augustNotes.ppt

66 http://www.thedoctorwithin.com/sugar/sugar-the-sweet-thief-of-life/

67 J Hepatol 2008;48:983–92.

68 *Nutr Res.* 2012 Sep;32(9):637-47.

69 Nutrition News and Views - Judith DeCava, C.C.N., L.N.C. Vol 3, no. 3.,"The Real Truth About Vitamins and Antioxidants"

70 http://cristivlad.com/energy-levels-under-ketosis-fats-carbs-and-atp/

71 Smith, M.A., and F. Lifshitz, "Excess fruit juice consumption as a contributing factor in nonorganic failure to thrive." Pediatrics 93, (1994):438-443.

72 http://www.alz.org/facts/

73 https://news.usc.edu/63669/fasting-triggers-stem-cell-regeneration-of-damaged-old-immune-system/

74 http://www.seattlepi.com/national/article/The-lowdown-on-topsoil-It-s-disappearing-1262214.php

75 http://www.scientificamerican.com/article/only-60-years-of-farming-left-if-soil-degradation-continues/

[76] http://www.seattlepi.com/national/article/The-lowdown-on-topsoil-It-s-disappearing-1262214.php

[77] Kesten, Deborah; Graham, Gray; Scherwitz, Larry (2011-06-06). Pottenger's Prophecy: How Food Resets Genes for Wellness or Illness

[78] https://monsanto.com/company/media/statements/agent-orange-background/

[79] Redfern, Robert, *The 'Miracle' Enzyme is Serrapeptase* pg. 13

[80] Am J Clin Nutr 2002, 76:1249–1255. Eur J Clin Nutr 2007, 61:355–361. Gut Pathog 2009, 1:6

[81] Bown, Stephen R. 2003 *SCURVY: HOW A SURGEON, A MARINER, AND A GENTLEMAN SOLVED THE GREATEST MEDICAL MYSTERY OF THE AGE OF SAIL*

[82] Mackowiak PA. Recycling Metchnikoff: Probiotics, the Intestinal Microbiome and the Quest for Long Life. *Frontiers in Public Health*. 2013;1:52. doi:10.3389/fpubh.2013.00052.

[83] Ken Inweregbu, BSc FRCA Jayshree Dave, MSc MRC Path MD MBA Alison Pittard, FRCA Contin Educ Anaesth Crit Care Pain (2005) 5 (1): 14-17.

[84] Xu M-Q, Cao H-L, Wang W-Q, et al. Fecal microbiota transplantation broadening its application beyond intestinal disorders. *World Journal of Gastroenterology : WJG*. 2015;21(1): 102-111. doi:10.3748/wjg.v21.i1.102.

[85] International Journal of Food Microbiology. Volume 146, Issue 2, 30 March 2011, Pages 144–150. Force M, Sparks WS, Ronzio RA. Phytother Res. 2000 May

[86] Butterfield, N. J. (2009). "Oxygen, animals and oceanic ventilation: An alternative view". *Geobiology*. **7** (1): 1–7. doi: 10.1111/j.1472-4669.2009.00188.x. PMID 19200141.

[87] Zimmer, Carl (3 October 2013). "Earth's Oxygen: A Mystery Easy to Take for Granted". *New York Times*. Retrieved 3 October 2013

[88] BC Wolverton; WL Douglas; K Bounds (July 1989). A study of interior landscape plants for indoor air pollution abatement (Report). NASA. NASA-TM-108061.

[89] Wasserman AJ, Patterson JL. THE CEREBRAL VASCULAR RESPONSE TO REDUCTION IN ARTERIAL CARBON DIOXIDE TENSION. *Journal of Clinical Investigation*. 1961;40(7):1297-1303.

[90] http://www.cbsnews.com/news/cdc-80-percent-of-american-adults-dont-get-recommended-exercise/

[91] http://www.nytimes.com/2011/04/17/magazine/mag-17sitting-t.html

[92] Kohlstadt, Ingrid, "Scientific Evidence for Musculoskeletal, Bariatric, and Sports Nutrition", page 30, published January 2006

[93] http://www.nytimes.com/2009/12/08/business/energy-environment/08water.html

[94] https://www.usatoday.com/story/news/2016/12/13/broken-system-means-millions-of-rural-americans-exposed-to-poisoned-or-untested-water/94071732/

[95] Moss, Brian (2008). "Water Pollution by Agriculture" (PDF). *Phil. Trans. Royal Society B*. **363**: 659–666. doi:10.1098/rstb.2007.2176.

[96] "Harmful Algal Bloom Management and Response: Assessment and Plan", Office of Science and Technology Policy, Sept. 2008

[97] http://www.mercola.com/downloads/bonus/chlorine/default.htm

98 http://www.waterbenefitshealth.com/chlorine-in-drinking-water.html

99 6 February 2000: [UK News] Parents told to sue for school drinking water 17 January 1999: [UK News] Water firms seek legal

100 *Fluoride*, Volume 14. No. 3, July 1981

101 European Commission. 2011. Critical review of any new evidence on the hazard profile, health effects, and human exposure to fluoride and the fluoridating agents of drinking water. Scientific Committee on Health and Environmental Risks (SCHER), page 4.

102 Cheng KK, Chalmers I, Sheldon TA. Adding fluoride to water supplies. BMJ : *British Medical Journal*. 2007;335(7622): 699-702. doi:10.1136/bmj.39318.562951.BE.

103 "Recommendations for Using Fluoride to Prevent and Control Dental Caries in the United States". August 17, 2001 / 50(RR14);1-42. https://www.cdc.gov/mmwr/preview/mmwrhtml/rr5014a1.htm

104 John Yiamouyiannis, *Fluoride*, 1990, Vol. 23, pp. 55-67

105 Kuopio, Finland —Ceased in 1993 owing to health studies (Caries Research 34: 462-468, 2000).
British Columbia, Canada-Ceased in 1993 (Community Dentistry and Oral Epidemiology 29: 37-47, 2001).

Chemnitz and Plauen, Germany-Ceased in 1993 (Community Dentistry and Oral Epidemiology 28: 382-9, 2000).

La Salud, Cuba- Ceased in 1990 (Caries Research 34: 20-5, 2000).

106 *Journal of the Canadian Dental Association*, Vol. 59, Apr. 1993, p. 334.

107 *JAMA*, Vol. 264, July 25, 1990, pp. 500

[108] Cooper et al., *JAMA*, Vol. 266, July 24, 1991, pp. 513-14.

[109] Christa Danielson et al., "Hip fractures and fluoridation in Utah's elderly population," *JAMA*, Vol. 268, Aug. 12, 1992, pp. 746-48.

[110] R.H. Belfast eat al., "Coronary Heart Disease. Differential Hemodynamics, Metabolic and Electrocardiographic Effects in Subjects with and without Angina during Atrial Pacing," *Circulation* 42, no. 4 (October 1970): 601-610, http://www.ncbi.nlm.nih.gov/pubmed/11993300.

[111] *EUROPEAN JOURNAL OF CANCER* 42 (2006) 2222–2232

[112] http://www.cancernetwork.com/articles/breast-cancer-risk-appears-fall-greater-sun-exposure

[113] https://www.sciencedaily.com/releases/2014/08/140806161659.htm

[114] https://www.cancer.org/cancer/skin-cancer/prevention-and-early-detection/what-is-uv-radiation.html

[115] Ikonomov et al. 1994, *Fukada* 2002.

[116] https://www.sciencedaily.com/releases/2007/03/070305202936.htm

[117] *Wilk v. American Medical Ass'n*, 671 F. Supp. 1465, N.D. Ill. 1987

[118] http://rotunda.upress.virginia.edu/founders/TSJN.html

[119] Hammond, Aaron, *Cannabis, Cannabinoids And The Benefits Of Medical Marijuana*, Kindle Edition, LOC - 216 of 604

① Mind

② Diet. 1st - 21 day reset
     3rd.

③ Digestion - 1st Mineral/Vitamins - Fulvic Humans _____
           3rd.   - Iodine _____
                                       - Zinc _____
                                       - Calci/Magn.

Made in the USA
San Bernardino, CA
21 February 2018